AN ATLAS of _

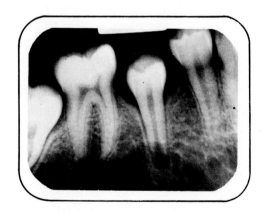 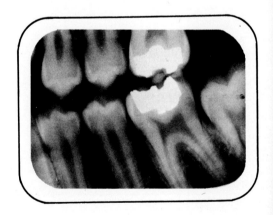

DENTAL RADIOGRAPHIC ANATOMY

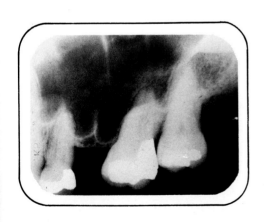

MYRON J. KASLE, D.D.S., M.S.D.

CHAIRMAN,
Department of Dental Radiology
Indiana University School of Dentistry
Indianapolis, Indiana

W. B. SAUNDERS COMPANY Philadelphia, London, Toronto

W. B. Saunders Company: West Washington Square
                           Philadelphia, PA   19105

                           1 St. Anne's Road
                           Eastbourne, East Sussex BN21 3UN, England

                           1 Goldthorne Avenue
                           Toronto, Ontario M8Z 5T9, Canada

Listed here is the latest translated edition of this book together with the
language of the translation and the publisher.   1st ed.   1/23/79
French   Masson Editeur   Paris, France

Listed here is the latest translated edition of this book together with the
language of the translation and the publisher.   1st ed.   6/19/79
Japanese   The Shorin Company Ltd., Tokyo, Japan

Listed here is the latest translated edition of this book together with the
language of the translation and the publisher.   1/E   7-25-79
Portugueses   Editora Interamericana Ltda. Rio de Janeiro, Brazil

Library of Congress Cataloging in Publication Data

Kasle, Myron J.

An atlas of dental radiographic anatomy.

Includes index.

1. Teeth — Radiography — Atlases.   2. Skull — Radiography —
   Atlases.   I. Title.

RK309.K37   617.6'07'572   76–20937

ISBN 0–7216–5294–8

An Atlas of Dental Radiographic Anatomy   ISBN   0-7216-5294-8

Last digit is the print number: 9   8   7   6

TO MY WIFE JUDY
AND SONS MICHAEL AND RICHARD

FOREWORD

In the field of dental radiology, we are witnessing the revitalization of interest in the intraoral and extraoral techniques, as well as in the interpretation of high quality films. Two reasons for this renewal of interest are the increased importance that is given to the need for complete preoperative records, and the realization that accurate and thorough interpretation of radiographs is essential to the development of a comprehensive treatment plan for the dental patient.

If this Atlas is studied by the reader in a careful and systematic manner, beginning with the illustrations of radiographs of the maxillary molar region and going to the illustrations of all segments of both arches and surrounding tissues, he or she will be provided with an excellent review of anatomic landmarks. It is also possible for the reader to open the book to any page and, in a few minutes, be reminded of important observations that affect treatment planning and dental practice. This Atlas will be a valuable addition to the library of all dental practitioners and dental auxiliaries. It will be especially useful to the dental student who is just becoming acquainted with the difficult task of learning radiographic interpretation. The individual interested in Forensic Dentistry will find it a valuable reference book, too.

This outstanding book is an unusually fine and unique contribution to dentistry and specifically to effective radiographic interpretation and utilization.

Ralph E. McDonald, D.D.S.

Dean, School of Dentistry
Indiana University

PREFACE

For a number of years, I have been encouraged by colleagues and students to produce an atlas of dental radiographs. The result is this Atlas. The dentist, dental student, hygienist and assistant will find that the radiographic images pictured have been lettered to indicate the areas of interest. The page facing each plate contains a legend that will enable the reader to make immediate identifications. It will be noted that the emphasis is placed on intraoral radiographs; however, several extraoral films have also been included. It is hoped that all who use this Atlas will find it helpful either in the complex everyday practice of dentistry or in classroom studies.

The author wishes to thank all those who have participated in producing this Atlas. For the production of the excellent photographic materials, thanks go to Mr. Richard Scott, Director of the Illustrations Department at Indiana University School of Dentistry and his staff consisting of Mike Halloran and Ellana Fears. Many thanks to the following members of the school's Radiology Department for their cooperation: Carol Ann Steinmetz, for typing the manuscript, and Dr. Jim Cottone, Gail Williamson, R.D.H., Isabell Poor and Rosalie Pollack.

Appreciation is also extended to Dr. Ralph E. McDonald, Dean of Indiana University School of Dentistry, whose encouragement has made this project possible.

CONTENTS

section one

INTRAORAL RADIOGRAPHS

Plate 1   MAXILLARY MOLAR REGION VIEW _____

A.   Maxillary tuberosity
B.   Floor of maxillary sinus
C.   Zygomatic process
D.   Maxillary sinus
E.   Zygomatic arch
F.   Shadow of soft tissue
G.   Film identification dot
H.   Coronoid process of mandible
I.   Alveolar ridge
J.   Retained roots
K.   Pterygoid plate
L.   Palatal root of permanent second molar
M.   Mesiobuccal root of permanent first molar
N.   Overlapping of tooth contacts
O.   Floor of nasal fossa
P.   Septum in maxillary sinus
Q.   Hamulus or hamular process
R.   Groove in maxillary sinus wall for superior alveolar nerve and vessels
S.   Microdont
T.   Distal surface of permanent second bicuspid
U.   Artifact caused by fixer contamination

Plate 1   MAXILLARY MOLAR REGION VIEW

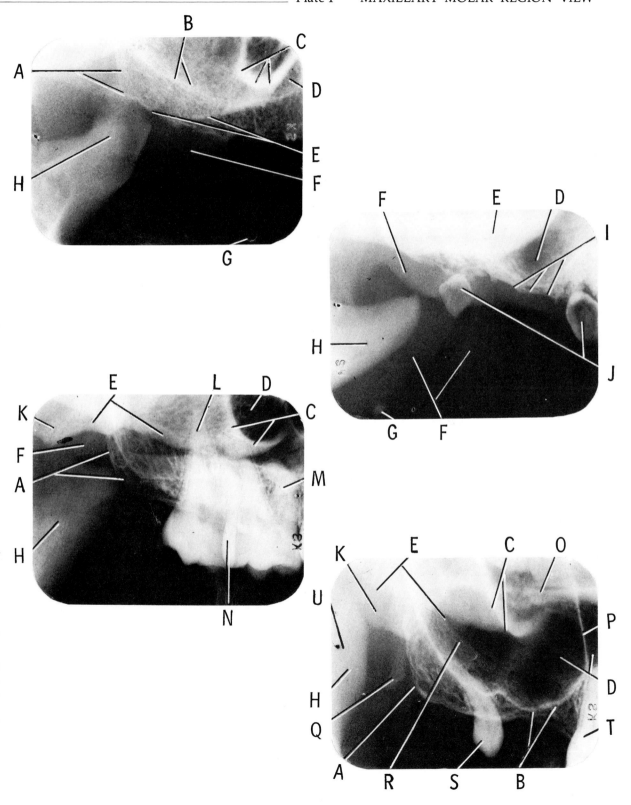

Plate 2   MAXILLARY MOLAR REGION VIEW _____

A.   Zygomatic process
B.   Maxillary sinus
C.   Posterior wall of maxillary sinus
D.   Hamular notch
E.   Maxillary tuberosity
F.   Coronoid process of mandible
G.   Lower border of zygomatic arch
H.   Palatal root of maxillary permanent first bicuspid
I.   Buccal root of maxillary permanent first bicuspid
J.   Distobuccal root of maxillary permanent first molar
K.   Mesiobuccal root of maxillary permanent first molar
L.   Dilacerated root of maxillary permanent second bicuspid
M.   Periapical radiolucency of maxillary permanent bicuspid
N.   Periapical radiolucency and buccal bone resorption of maxillary permanent first molar

Plate 2   MAXILLARY MOLAR REGION VIEW

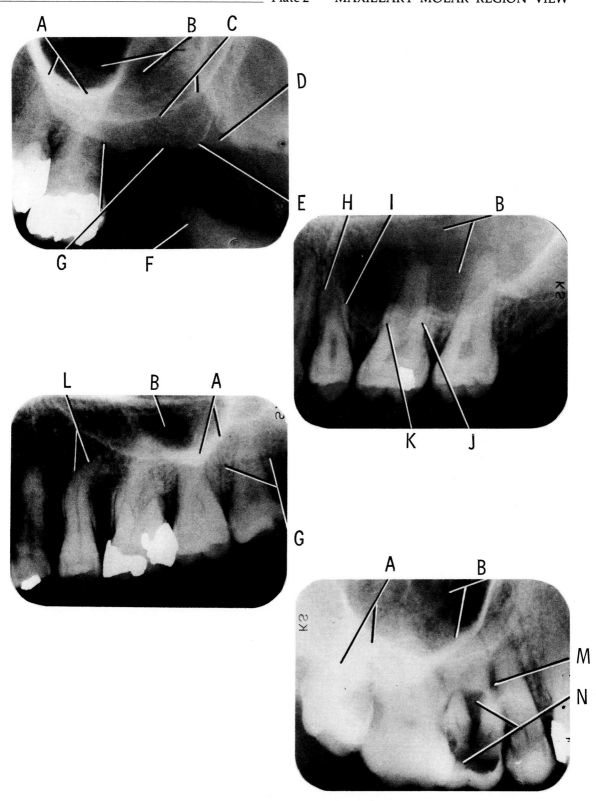

Plate 3   MAXILLARY MOLAR REGION VIEW _____

A.   Coronoid process of mandible
B.   Microdont
C.   Healed extraction site
D.   Maxillary sinus
E.   Unerupted maxillary permanent third molar
F.   Follicle of maxillary permanent third molar
G.   Hamulus—medial pterygoid plate
H.   Zygomatic process

Plate 3   MAXILLARY MOLAR REGION VIEW

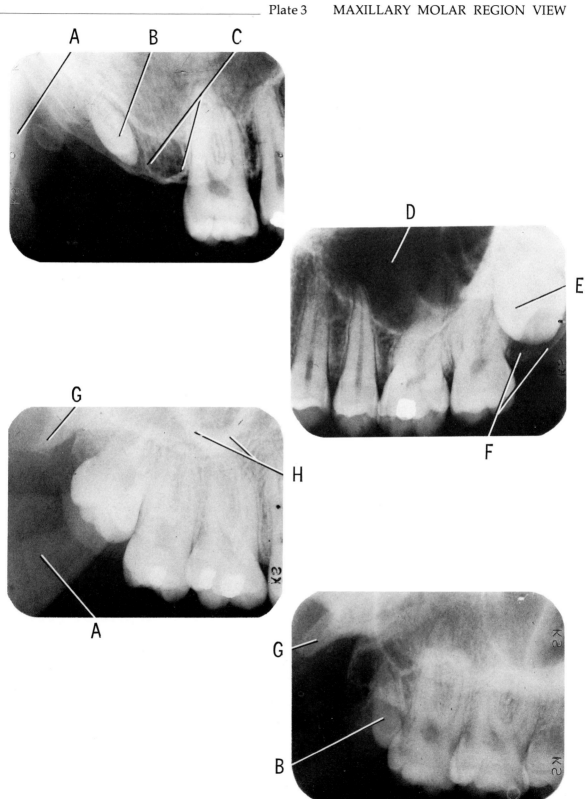

Plate 4   MAXILLARY MOLAR REGION VIEW _____

A.   Lower border of zygomatic arch
B.   Maxillary sinus
C.   Maxillary tuberosity
D.   Sclerotic bone
E.   Maxillary sinus depression
F.   Zygomatic process
G.   Lateral pterygoid plate
H.   Hamulus — medial pterygoid plate
I.   Coronoid process of mandible
J.   Film identification dot
K.   Floor of maxillary sinus
L.   Nutrient canal in maxillary sinus wall
M.   Soft tissue covering maxillary tuberosity
N.   Sequestrum from previous extraction

Plate 4   MAXILLARY MOLAR REGION VIEW

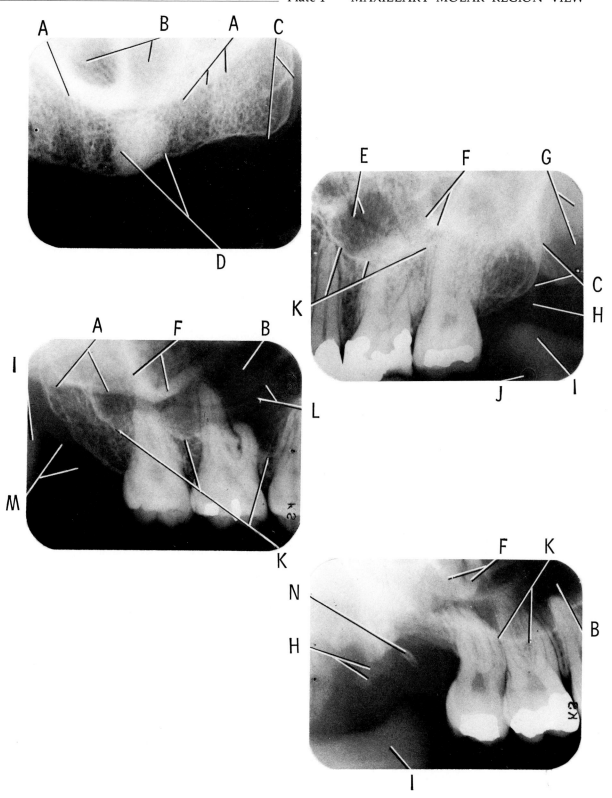

Plate 5   MAXILLARY MOLAR REGION VIEW _____

A.   Nasal fossa
B.   Floor of nasal fossa
C.   Maxillary sinus
D.   Floor of maxillary sinus
E.   Mesiobuccal root of maxillary permanent first molar
F.   Distobuccal root of maxillary permanent first molar
G.   Palatal root of maxillary permanent first molar
H.   Endodontic treatment in root of maxillary permanent second bicuspid
I.   Recurrent caries under gold crown of maxillary permanent first molar
J.   Coronoid process of mandible
K.   Film identification dot
L.   Zygomatic process
M.   Nutrient canal in maxillary sinus wall

Plate 5   MAXILLARY MOLAR REGION VIEW

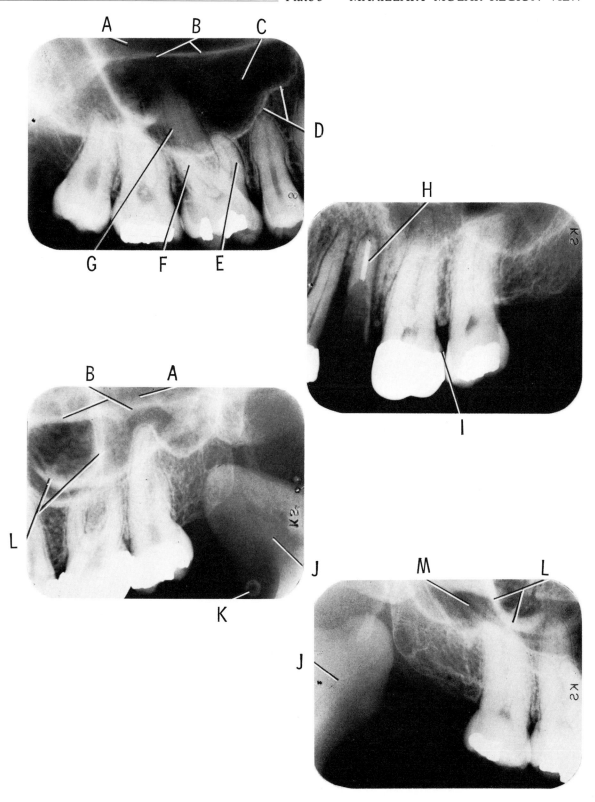

Plate 6   MAXILLARY MOLAR REGION VIEW _____

A.   Lateral pterygoid plate
B.   Hamulus—medial pterygoid plate
C.   Film identification dot
D.   Coronoid process of mandible
E.   Maxillary sinus
F.   Zygomatic process
G.   Soft tissue shadow
H.   Thin plate of bone distal to maxillary third molar
I.   Impacted maxillary permanent third molar
J.   Soft tissue over maxillary third molar
K.   Impacted supernumerary molar
L.   Chrome steel orthodontic band

Plate 6   MAXILLARY MOLAR REGION VIEW

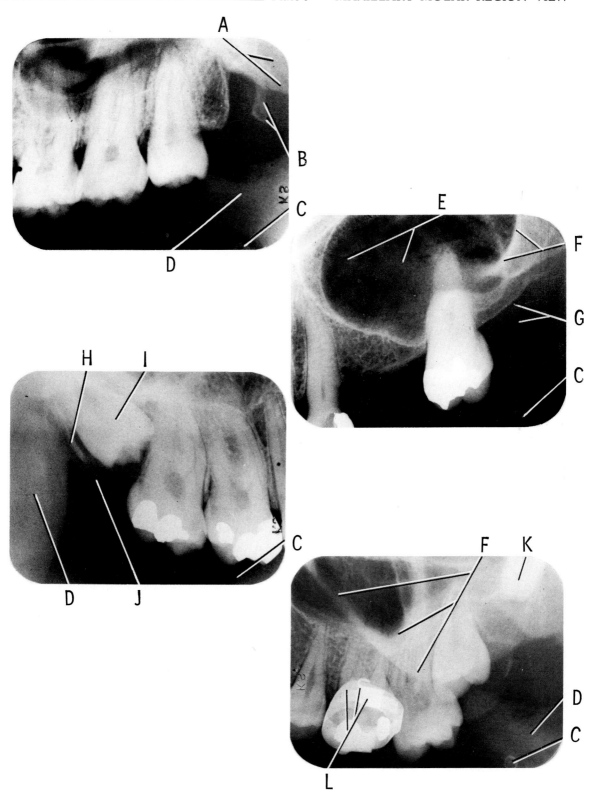

Plate 7   MAXILLARY BICUSPID REGION VIEW _____

A.   Unerupted maxillary permanent first molar
B.   Unerupted maxillary permanent second bicuspid
C.   Unerupted maxillary permanent first bicuspid
D.   Unerupted maxillary permanent cuspid
E.   Partially resorbed root of maxillary primary cuspid
F.   Maxillary primary first molar
G.   Maxillary primary second molar
H.   Radiolucent resin restoration
I.   Radiopaque metallic lingual restoration
J.   Endodontically treated maxillary permanent first bicuspid with retrograde metal restoration
K.   Gold post and core restoration
L.   Floor of nasal fossa
M.   Buccal root of maxillary permanent first bicuspid
N.   Palatal root of maxillary permanent first bicuspid
O.   Nutrient canal in maxillary sinus wall

Plate 7   MAXILLARY BICUSPID REGION VIEW

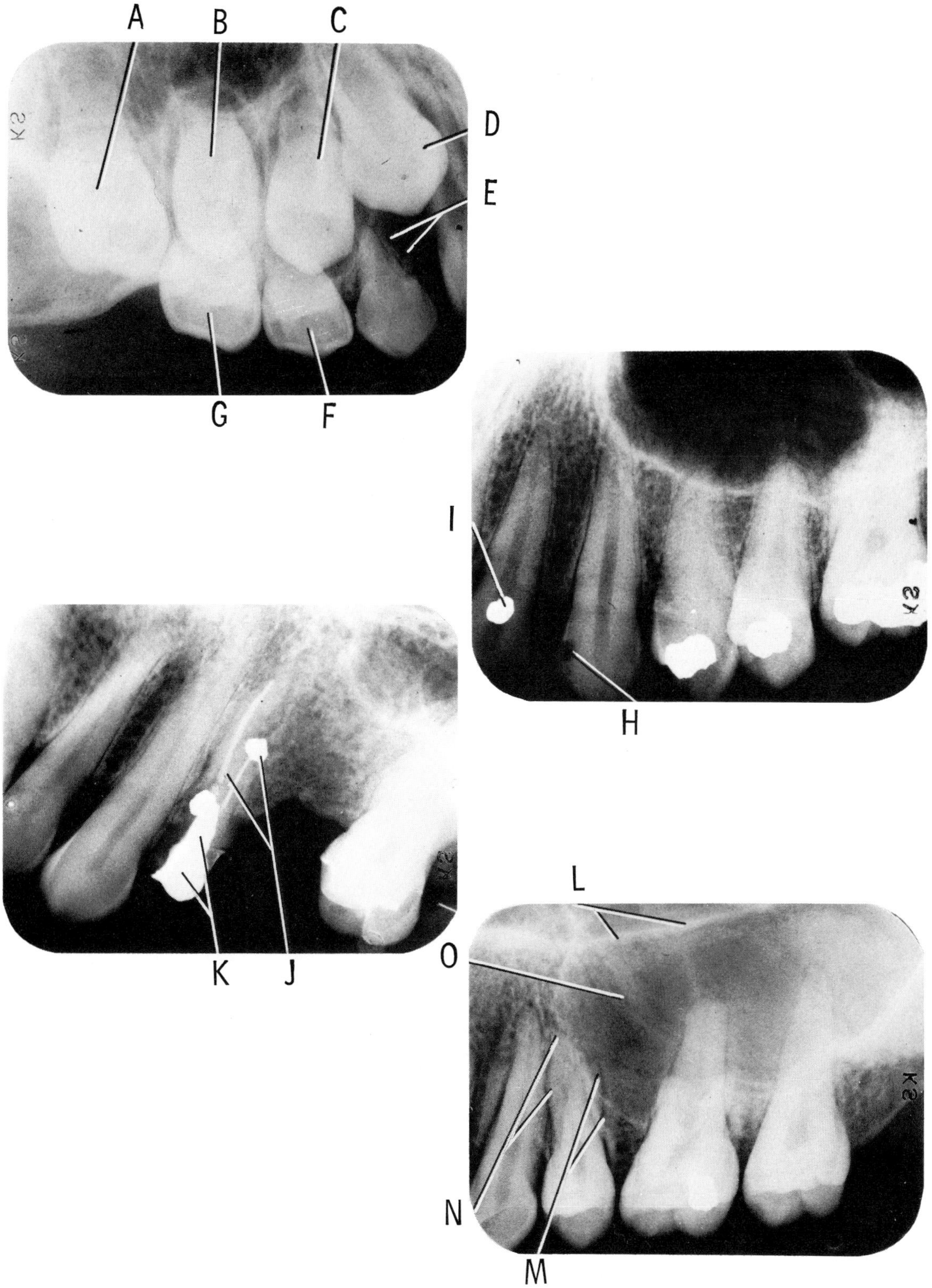

Plate 8   MAXILLARY BICUSPID REGION VIEW _____

A.   Zygomatic process
B.   Maxillary sinus
C.   Oroantral fistula
D.   Supernumerary tooth
E.   Film crease
F.   Septum in maxillary sinus
G.   Sclerosed pulp chambers
H.   Resorbed bone of edentulous arch
I.   Floor of nasal fossa
J.   Cusp of mandibular permanent first molar
K.   Maxillary primary second molar
L.   Maxillary primary first molar
M.   Maxillary primary cuspid

Plate 8   MAXILLARY BICUSPID REGION VIEW

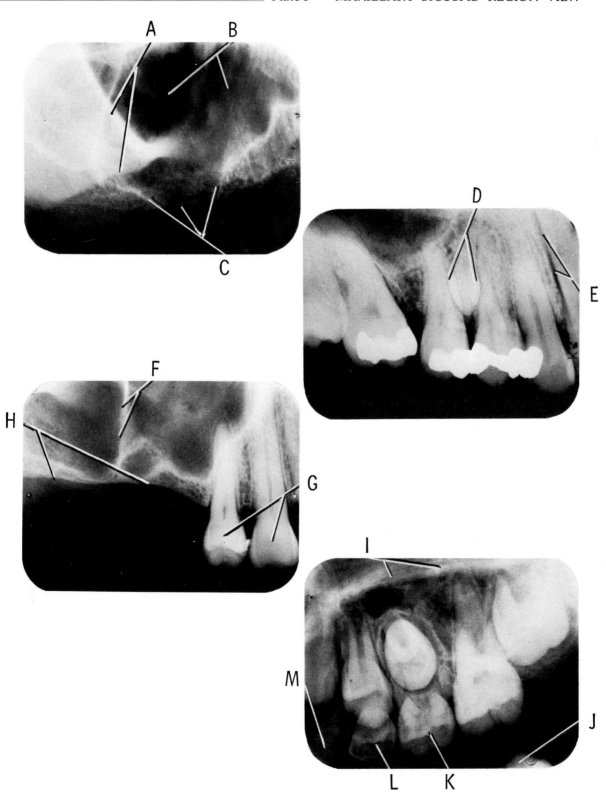

Plate 9   MAXILLARY BICUSPID REGION VIEW _____

- **A.** Maxillary sinus
- **B.** Zygoma
- **C.** Groove of nutrient canal in maxillary sinus
- **D.** Remnant of retained root tip
- **E.** Cervical burnout (adumbration)
- **F.** Septum in maxillary sinus
- **G.** Nasolabial fold
- **H.** Microdont
- **I.** Gold pontics
- **J.** Gold crown abutments

Plate 9   MAXILLARY BICUSPID REGION VIEW

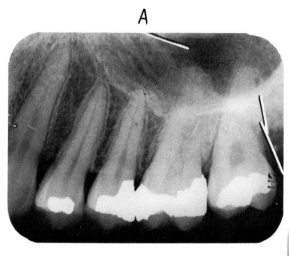

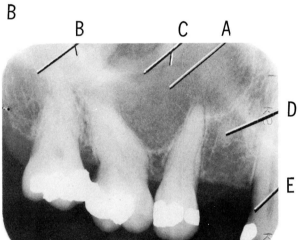

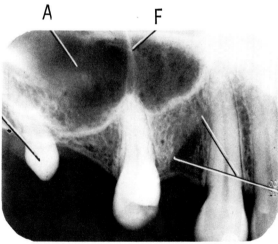

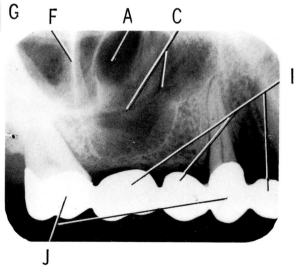

Plate 10   MAXILLARY BICUSPID REGION VIEW _____

A.   Floor of maxillary sinus
B.   Maxillary sinus
C.   Zygomatic process
D.   Carious lesions
E.   Septa in maxillary sinus
F.   Palatal root of maxillary permanent first molar
G.   Lower border of zygomatic arch
H.   Periapical radiolucency of mesial root, maxillary permanent first molar
I.   Gold crown abutment of maxillary permanent cuspid
J.   Gold pontics for maxillary bridge
K.   Gold crown abutment of maxillary permanent first molar
L.   Floor of nasal fossa

Plate 10   MAXILLARY BICUSPID REGION VIEW

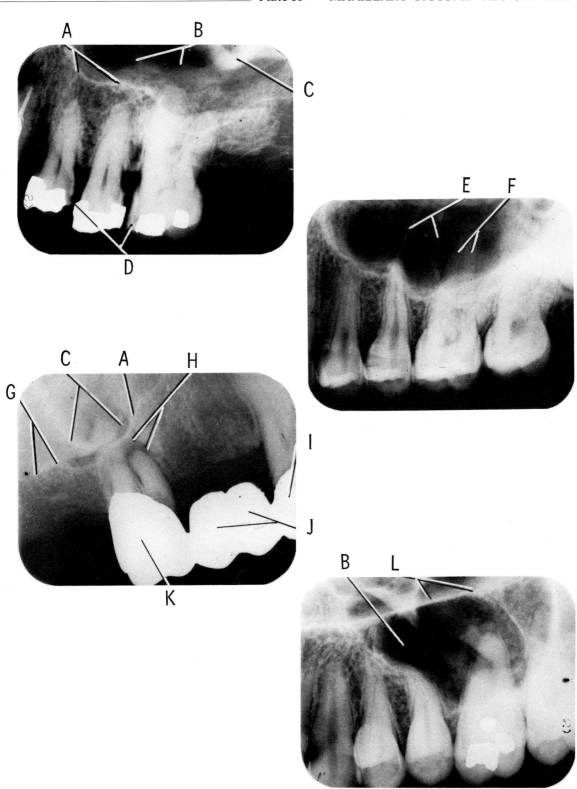

Plate 11   MAXILLARY BICUSPID–MOLAR REGION VIEW

A.   Maxillary sinus septum
B.   Palatal roots
C.   Maxillary tuberosity
D.   Area of bone resorption
E.   Heavy calculous deposits
F.   Compound odontoma
G.   Palatal cusp of maxillary permanent first bicuspid

Plate 11   MAXILLARY BICUSPID–MOLAR REGION VIEW

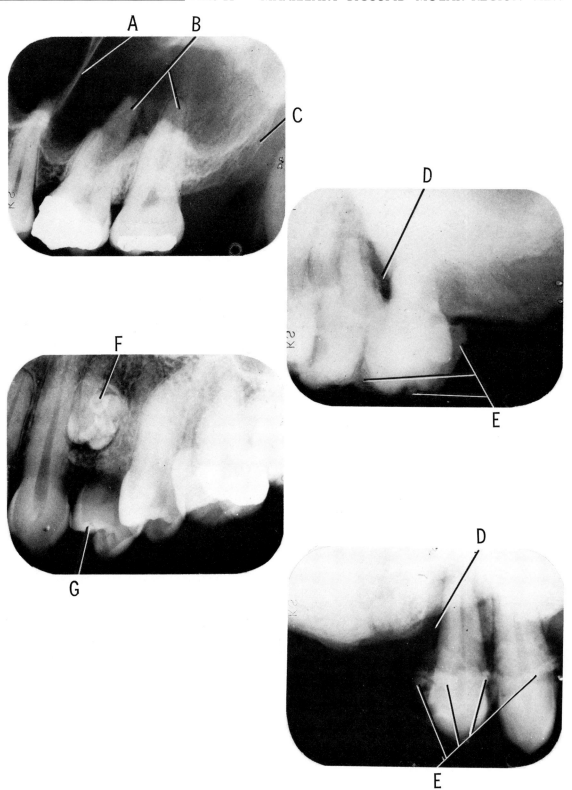

Plate 12   MAXILLARY CUSPID REGION VIEW _____

A.   Maxillary sinus
B.   Bone septum separating nasal fossa and maxillary sinus
C.   Nasal fossa
D.   Nasolabial fold
E.   Shadow of nose
F.   Cement base
G.   Resin restoration
H.   Gold post and core in endodontically treated tooth
I.   Periapical radiolucency in infected tooth
J.   Pulpally exposed tooth

Plate 12   MAXILLARY CUSPID REGION VIEW

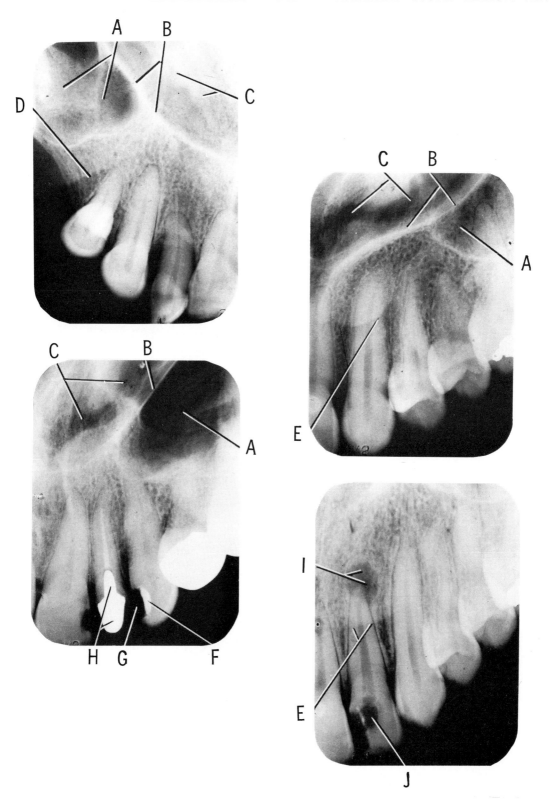

Plate 13   MAXILLARY CUSPID REGION VIEW

A.   Maxillary sinus
B.   Bone septum between nasal fossa and maxillary sinus
C.   Nasal fossa
D.   Radiolucent resin restorations
E.   Maxillary primary cuspid
F.   Maxillary primary first molar
G.   Nasal septum
H.   Carious lesion in maxillary permanent first bicuspid
I.   Radiopaque cement
J.   Crown prepared for jacket crown restoration
K.   Metal tubing post placed in pulp canal
L.   Carious lesion in maxillary permanent central incisor
M.   Periapical lesion due to metal tubing in pulp canal

Plate 13   MAXILLARY CUSPID REGION VIEW

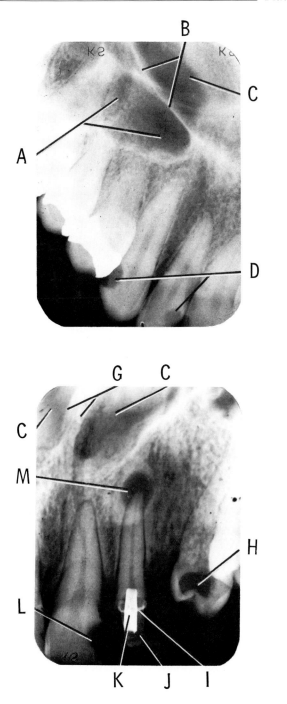

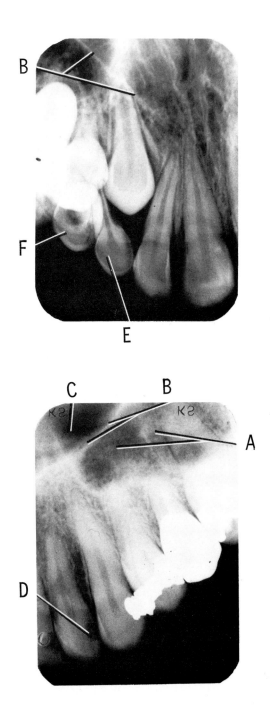

Plate 14   MAXILLARY CUSPID REGION VIEW _____

A.   Bone separating nasal fossa and maxillary sinus
B.   Nasal fossa
C.   Alveolus of recently extracted maxillary permanent lateral incisor
D.   Alveolus of recently extracted maxillary permanent central incisor
E.   Maxillary permanent cuspid
F.   Buccal cusp of maxillary permanent first bicuspid
G.   Palatal cusp of maxillary permanent first bicuspid
H.   Maxillary permanent second bicuspid
I.   Shadow of soft tissue of nose
J.   Floor of maxillary sinus
K.   Maxillary sinus
L.   Maxillary permanent central incisors
M.   Transposed maxillary permanent first bicuspid
N.   Transposed maxillary permanent cuspid
O.   Metal restorations
P.   Follicle of maxillary permanent cuspid
Q.   Incisive foramen
R.   Unerupted maxillary permanent cuspid
S.   Maxillary permanent lateral incisor
T.   Palatal cusp of maxillary permanent second bicuspid
U.   Buccal cusp of maxillary permanent second bicuspid
V.   Shadow of maxillary permanent first molar
W.   Septum in maxillary sinus
X.   Resin restorations
Y.   Film identification dot

Plate 14   MAXILLARY CUSPID REGION VIEW

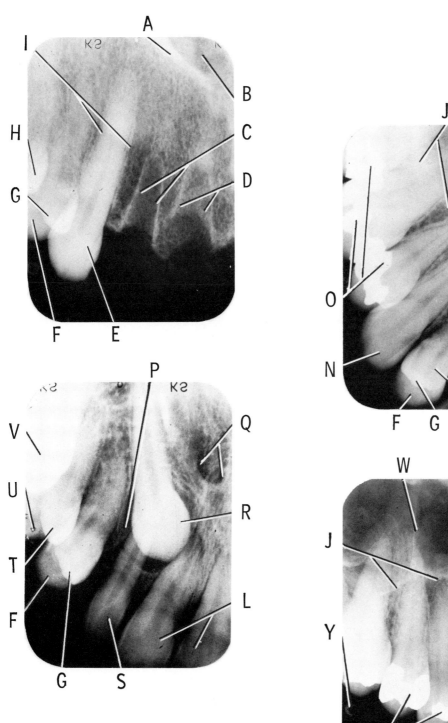

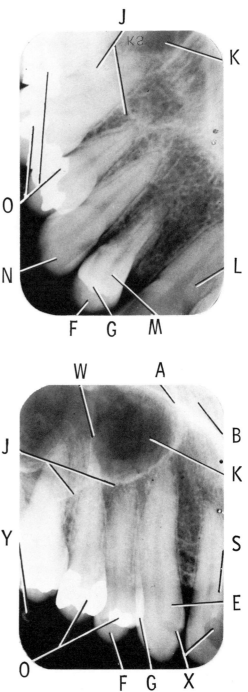

Plate 15   MAXILLARY CUSPID REGION VIEW _____

A.   Nasal fossa
B.   Floor of nasal fossa
C.   Maxillary sinus
D.   Floor of maxillary sinus
E.   Buccal root of maxillary permanent first bicuspid
F.   Palatal root of maxillary permanent first bicuspid
G.   Buccal cusp of maxillary permanent first bicuspid
H.   Resin restoration
I.   Cement base
J.   Metallic lingual restoration
K.   Film identification dot
L.   Shadow of maxillary permanent first bicuspid
M.   Overlapping contacts
N.   Periapical radiolucency around maxillary permanent first bicuspid
O.   Carious lesion
P.   Periapical radiolucency around maxillary permanent lateral incisor
Q.   Palatal cusp of maxillary permanent second bicuspid
R.   Palatal cusp of maxillary permanent first bicuspid
S.   Resorbed root of maxillary permanent lateral incisor

Plate 15   MAXILLARY CUSPID REGION VIEW

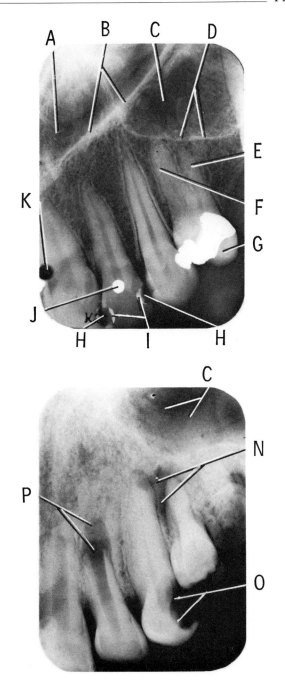

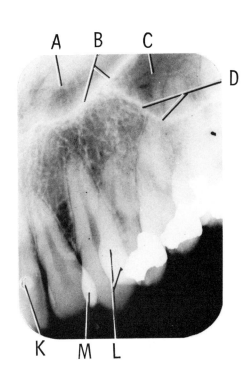

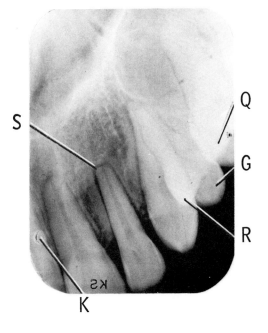

Plate 16   MAXILLARY INCISOR REGION VIEW

A.   Maxillary primary lateral incisor
B.   Unerupted maxillary permanent lateral incisor
C.   Developing root of erupting maxillary permanent central incisor
D.   Nasal fossa
E.   Nasal septum
F.   Median palatal suture
G.   Crowns of maxillary primary central incisors with resorbed roots
H.   Anterior nasal spine
I.   Mesiodens
J.   Opening made on lingual side of tooth for attempted endodontic treat-
      ment
K.   Erosion
L.   Endodontic filling material
M.   Silver alloy retrograde filling
N.   Resin restorations

Plate 16   MAXILLARY INCISOR REGION VIEW

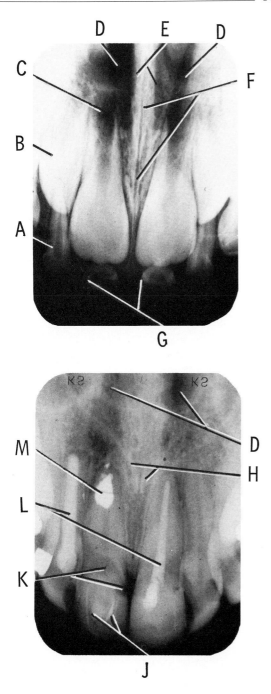

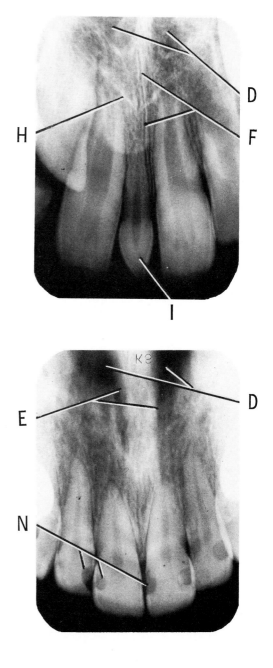

Plate 17   MAXILLARY INCISOR REGION VIEW _____

A.   Nasal fossa
B.   Nasal septum
C.   Anterior nasal spine
D.   Incisive foramen
E.   Lip line
F.   Lingual metal restoration
G.   Median palatal suture
H.   Film identification dot
I.   Anterior extent of maxillary sinus
J.   Carious lesion
K.   Gold pontic
L.   Gold crown restoration
M.   Surgical defect
N.   Soft tissue of nose

Plate 17   MAXILLARY INCISOR REGION VIEW

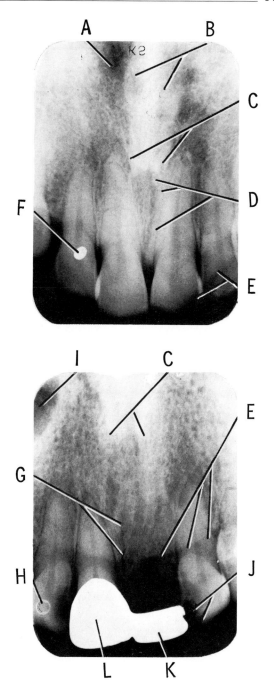

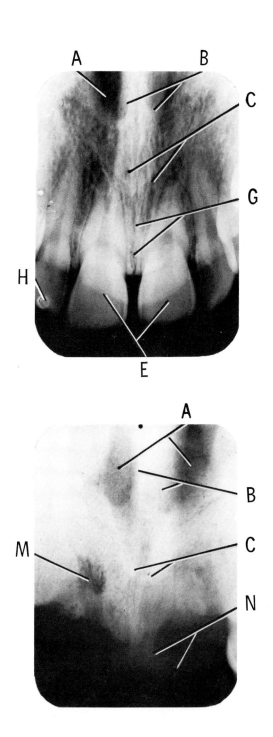

Plate 18   MAXILLARY INCISOR REGION VIEW

A.   Unerupted maxillary permanent cuspid
B.   Nasal septum
C.   Radiolucent line indicating cervical area and bone level
D.   Shadow of soft tissue of nose
E.   Gold pontics of anterior bridge
F.   Nasal fossa
G.   Supernumerary teeth
H.   Unerupted maxillary permanent lateral incisor
I.   Unerupted maxillary permanent central incisor
J.   Maxillary primary lateral incisor
K.   Maxillary primary central incisor

Plate 18   MAXILLARY INCISOR REGION VIEW

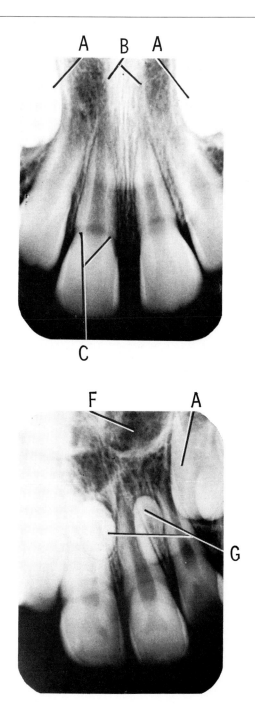

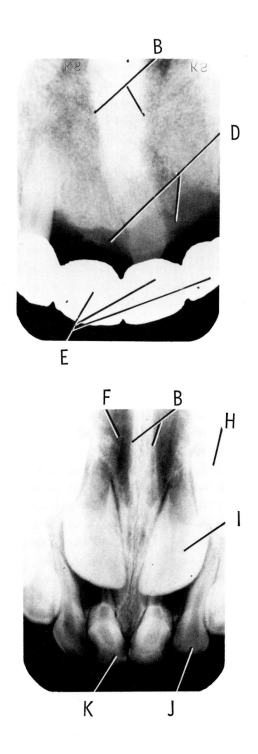

Plate 19   MAXILLARY INCISOR REGION VIEW

A. Nasal fossa
B. Anterior nasal spine
C. Carious lesion
D. Median palatal suture
E. Incisive nerve foramen
F. Periapical lesion
G. Carious lesion involving pulp chamber
H. Shadow of lip line
I. Supernumerary tooth (mesiodens)
J. Nasal septum
K. Developing roots of maxillary permanent central incisors
L. Crown remnants of maxillary primary lateral incisors

Plate 19   MAXILLARY INCISOR REGION VIEW

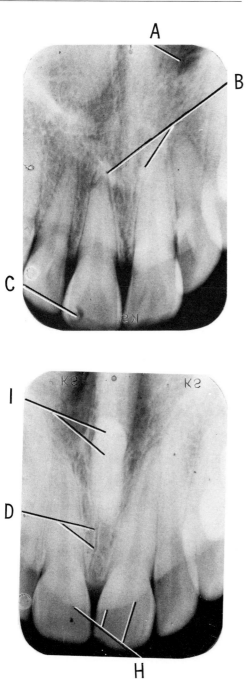

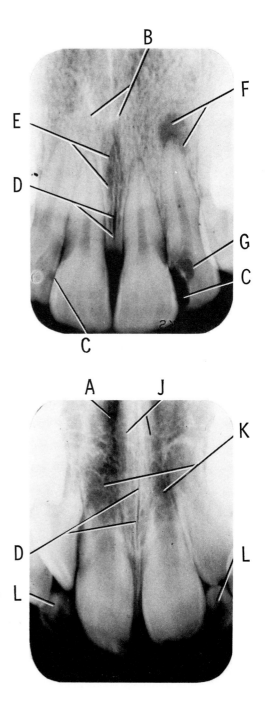

Plate 20   MAXILLARY INCISOR REGION VIEW _____

A. Impacted maxillary permanent central incisor
B. Nasal fossae
C. Incisal attrition
D. Resorbed root
E. Gold post and core of endodontically treated maxillary permanent central incisors
F. Reinforcing wire under resin restoration replacing fractured incisal edge
G. Overlapping of maxillary permanent lateral and central incisors
H. Crown fracture of maxillary permanent central incisor
I. Shadow of lip line

Plate 20   MAXILLARY INCISOR REGION VIEW

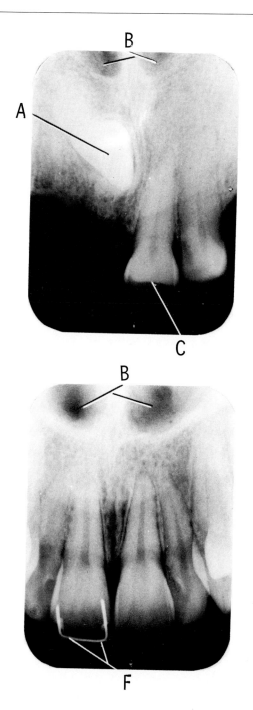

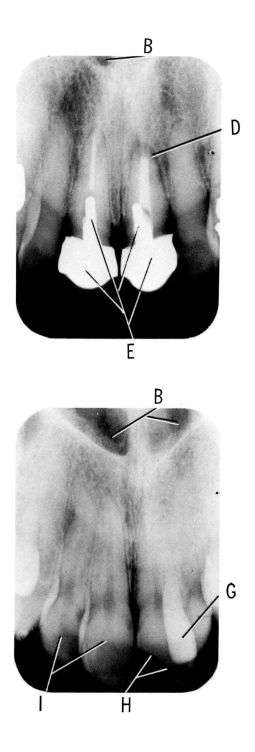

Plate 21   MAXILLARY INCISOR REGION VIEW _____

A.   Nasal conchae in nasal fossae
B.   Nasal fossae
C.   Anterior nasal spine
D.   Shadow of lip line
E.   Nasal septum
F.   Incisive nerve foramen
G.   Area of missing anterior restoration
H.   Carious lesion
I.   Median palatal suture
J.   Resorbed roots
K.   Resin restoration

Plate 21   MAXILLARY INCISOR REGION VIEW

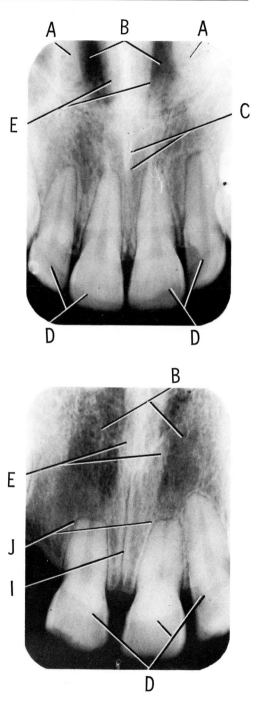

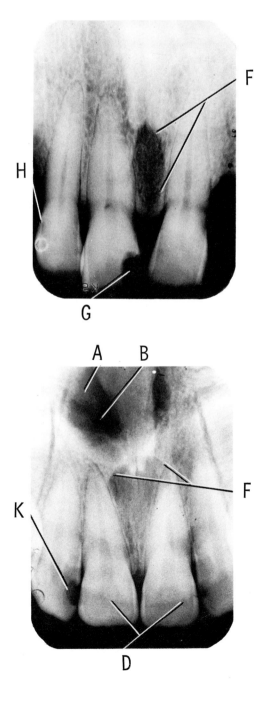

Plate 22   MAXILLARY INCISOR REGION VIEW _____

A.   Nasal fossa
B.   Nasal septum
C.   Film crease
D.   Impacted maxillary permanent cuspid
E.   Rubber material around metal film holder
F.   Metal film holder
G.   Soft tissue of nose
H.   Zinc oxide temporary restoration
I.   Anterior nasal spine
J.   Cement bases under resin restorations
K.   Carious lesion

Plate 22   MAXILLARY INCISOR REGION VIEW

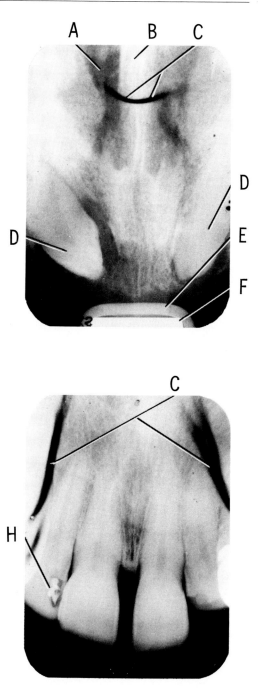

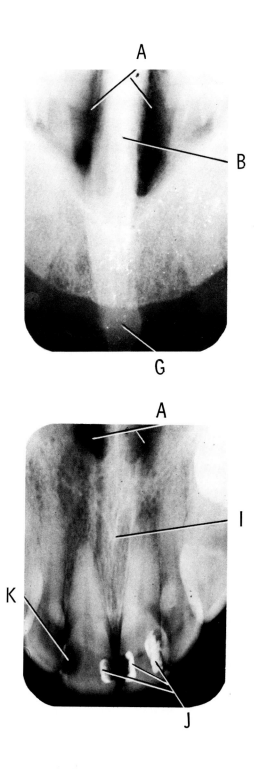

Plate 23   MANDIBULAR MOLAR REGION VIEW

A. Mandibular canal
B. Film identification dot
C. External oblique ridge
D. Cervical burnout (adumbration)
E. Enamel pearl
F. Internal oblique ridge
G. Overhanging restoration
H. Radiolucent normal bone area

Plate 23   MANDIBULAR MOLAR REGION VIEW

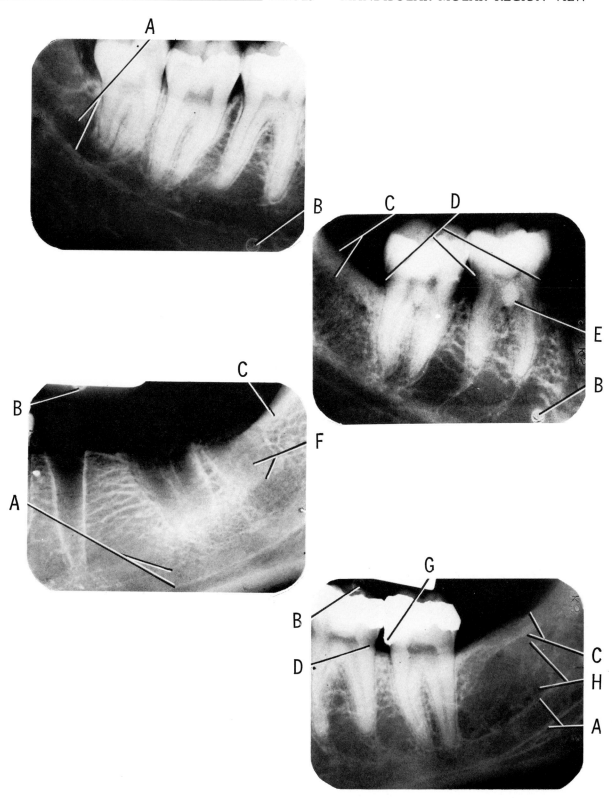

Plate 24   MANDIBULAR MOLAR REGION VIEW _____

A.   Recurrent caries
B.   Area of bone resorption
C.   Fused roots
D.   Dilacerated root
E.   Mandibular canal
F.   Healing extraction site

Plate 24   MANDIBULAR MOLAR REGION VIEW

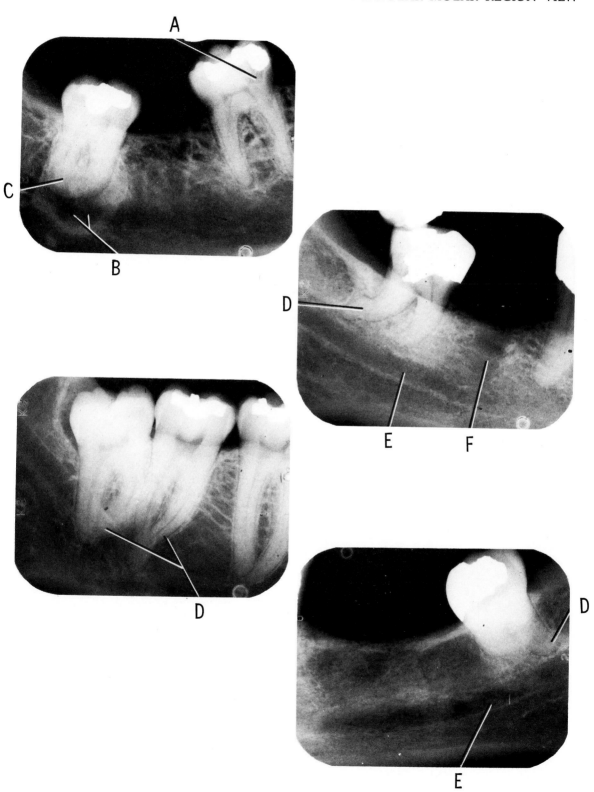

Plate 25   MANDIBULAR MOLAR REGION VIEW _____

A.   Pulp stone
B.   Retained root fragments
C.   Radiolucency indicating bone resorption
D.   Radiolucency indicating bone destruction due to periodontal disease
E.   Film identification dot
F.   Mandibular canal
G.   External oblique ridge
H.   Enamel pearl
I.   Cortical bone of inferior border of mandible
J.   Healing extraction site
K.   Tooth crown destruction due to caries
L.   Bone overlying developing permanent third molar
M.   Developing permanent third molar in follicle
N.   Early calcification of bifurcation of permanent third molar
O.   Periapical bone loss due to carious lesion
P.   Cervical burnout (adumbration)

Plate 25   MANDIBULAR MOLAR REGION VIEW

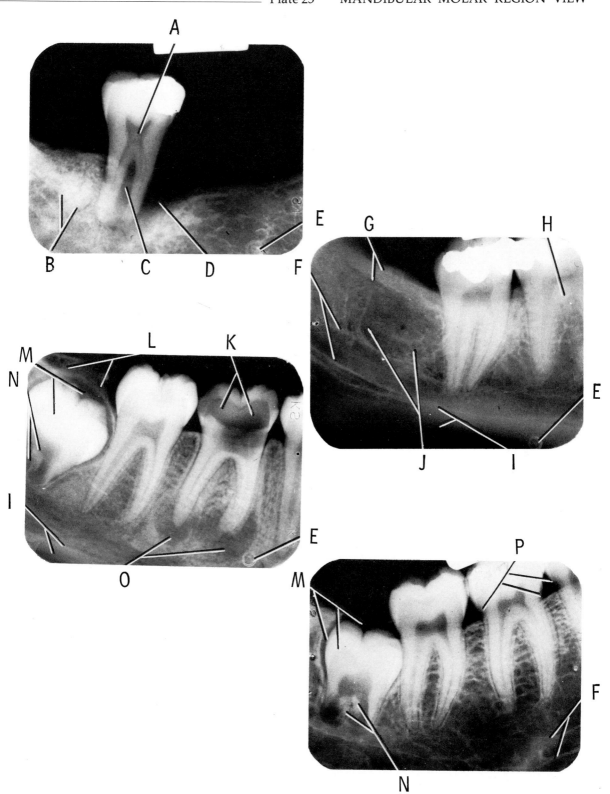

Plate 26   MANDIBULAR MOLAR REGION VIEW _____

A.   Lamina dura of tooth follicle
B.   Developing mandibular permanent third molar in follicle
C.   Alveolar bone level
D.   Developing roots of mandibular permanent second molar
E.   Horizontal developing mandibular permanent third molar
F.   Overhanging restoration
G.   Horizontally impacted mandibular permanent third molar

Plate 26   MANDIBULAR MOLAR REGION VIEW

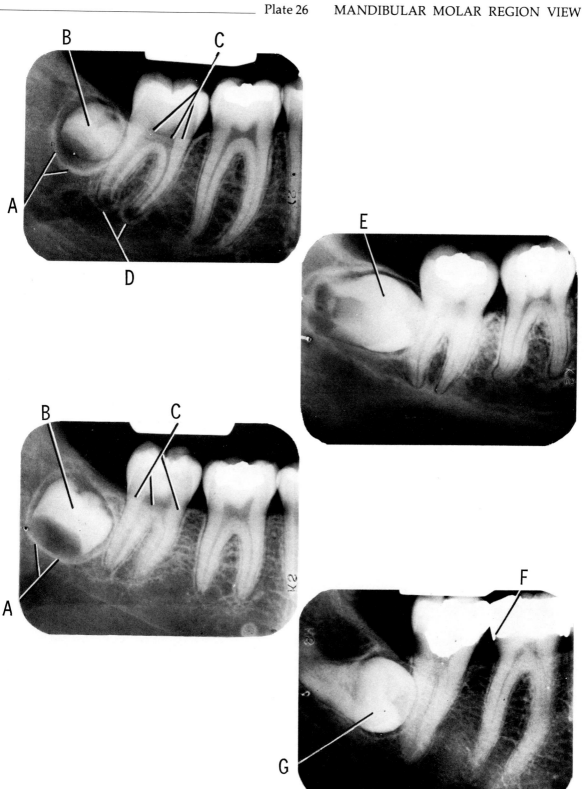

Plate 27   MANDIBULAR MOLAR REGION VIEW _____

A.   External oblique ridge
B.   Shadow of soft tissue
C.   Carious lesion in permanent third molar
D.   Portion of metal film holder
E.   Carious lesion in permanent second molar
F.   Normal bone trabeculation
G.   Retained root tip in soft tissue
H.   Distal surface of permanent second bicuspid
I.   Mandibular canal
J.   Film identification dot
K.   Radiolucent area indicating bone loss due to cariously infected tooth
L.   Lamina dura at alveolar bone crest
M.   Bone located over unerupted permanent third molar
N.   Unerupted developing permanent third molar located in developing
     tooth follicle
O.   Incompletely developed apices
P.   Periodontal ligament space (radiolucent line)
Q.   Cortical bone of inferior border of mandible
R.   Silver restoration
S.   Zinc phosphate cement base
T.   Gold full crown
U.   Distal root canal
V.   Interradicular bone
W.   Follicle of developing tooth
X.   Mesially impacted permanent third molar
Y.   Overlapping contacts of permanent molars
Z.   Apex of mesial root of permanent first molar

Plate 27   MANDIBULAR MOLAR REGION VIEW

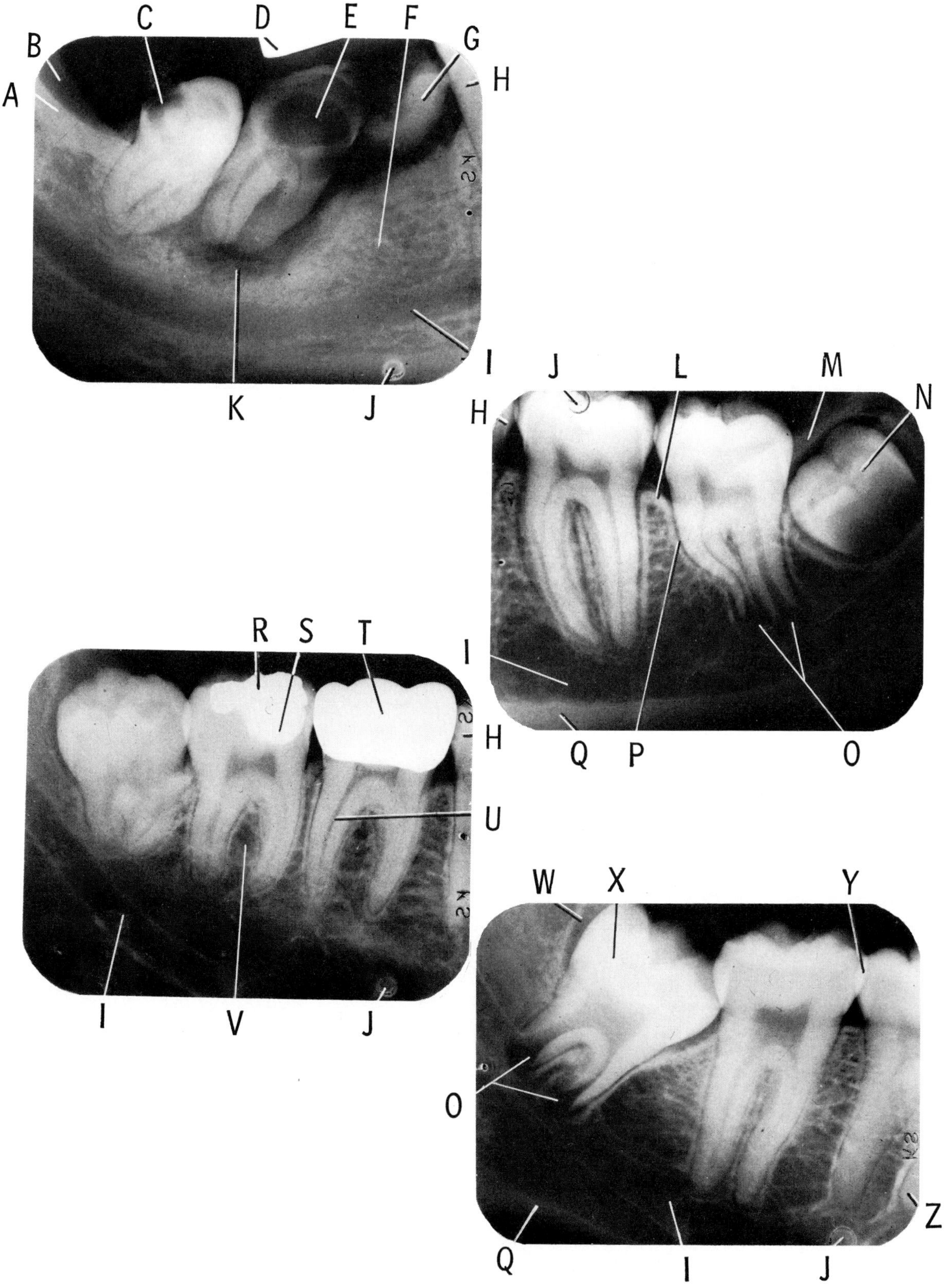

Plate 28   MANDIBULAR MOLAR REGION VIEW

A.   Distally impacted mandibular permanent third molar
B.   Medullary bone resorbed indicating possible cyst formation
C.   Mandibular canal
D.   Cortical bone of inferior border of mandible
E.   Internal oblique ridge
F.   Developing crown of mandibular permanent third molar
G.   Portion of metal film holder
H.   Film identification dot
I.   Rubber material surrounding film holder
J.   Resorbed roots of mandibular permanent first molar
K.   Bent corner of film

Plate 28   MANDIBULAR MOLAR REGION VIEW

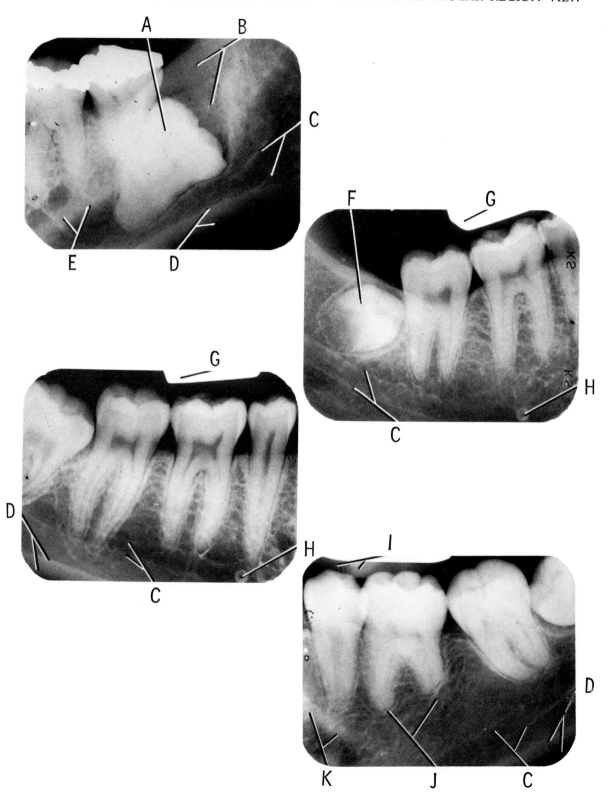

Plate 29   MANDIBULAR BICUSPID REGION VIEW _____

A.   Zinc phosphate cement base
B.   Silver restoration
C.   Cast gold restoration
D.   Portion of metal film holder
E.   Rubber material surrounding film holder
F.   Cervical burnout (adumbration)
G.   Bent corner of film
H.   Mental foramen
I.   Mandibular canal
J.   Alveolar bone ridge
K.   External oblique ridge
L.   Internal oblique ridge
M.   Submandibular fossa
N.   Cast gold crown bridge abutment
O.   Cast gold bridge pontics
P.   Healed extraction sites

Plate 29   MANDIBULAR BICUSPID REGION VIEW

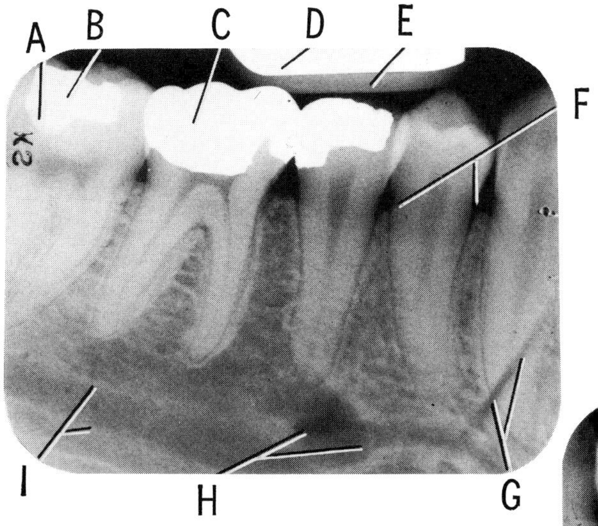

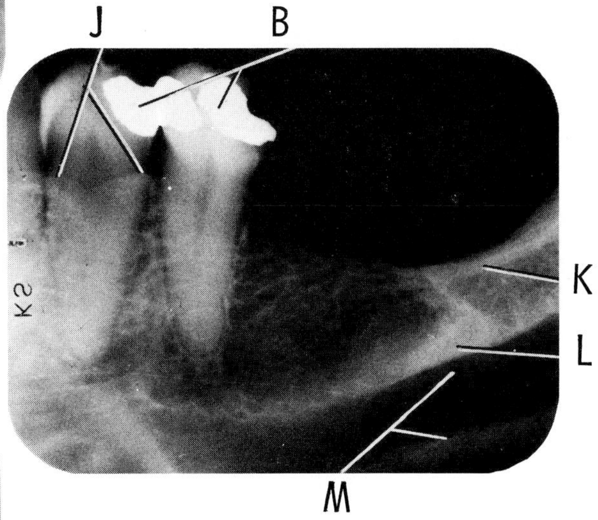

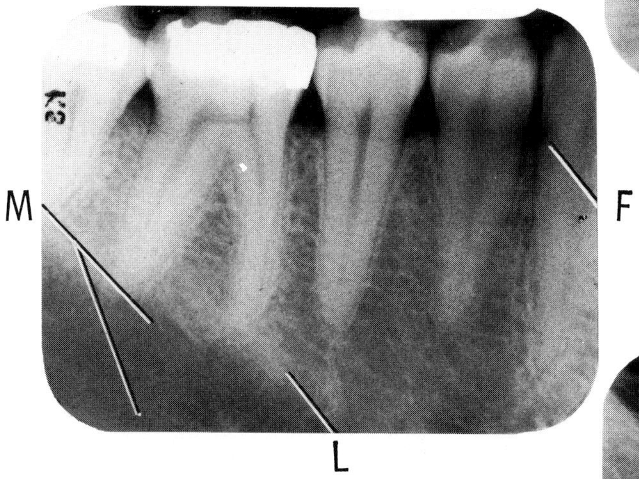

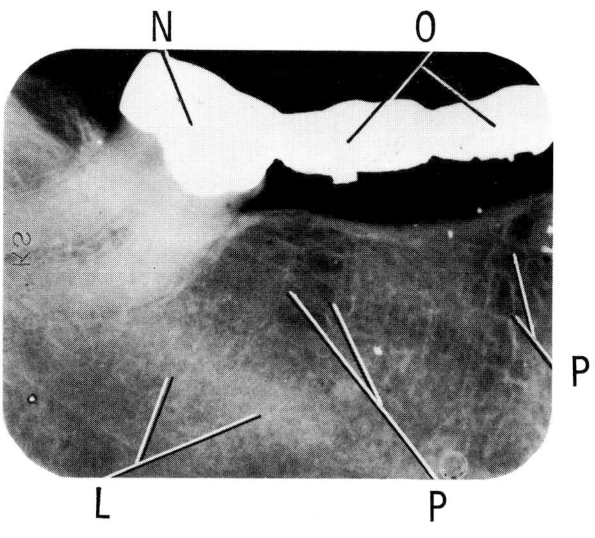

Plate 30   MANDIBULAR BICUSPID REGION VIEW _____

A.   Mandibular permanent cuspid
B.   Film identification dot
C.   Crown of resorbed mandibular primary first molar
D.   Mandibular primary second molar
E.   Erupting mandibular permanent second molar
F.   Incompletely developed roots of mandibular permanent first molar
G.   Developing crown of mandibular permanent second bicuspid
H.   Developing mandibular permanent first bicuspid
I.   Incompletely developed root of mandibular permanent first bicuspid
J.   Lingual cusp of mandibular permanent first bicuspid
K.   Portion of metal film holder
L.   Supernumerary mandibular bicuspid
M.   Submandibular fossa
N.   Dilacerated mesial root of mandibular permanent first molar
O.   Mental foramen
P.   Buccal cusps of mandibular permanent first molar
Q.   Unerupted mandibular permanent cuspid
R.   Lingual cusps of mandibular permanent first molar
S.   Follicle of developing permanent second molar

Plate 30   MANDIBULAR BICUSPID REGION VIEW

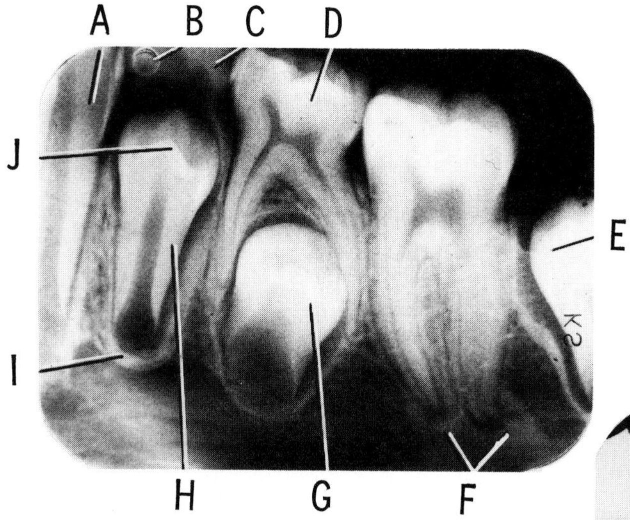

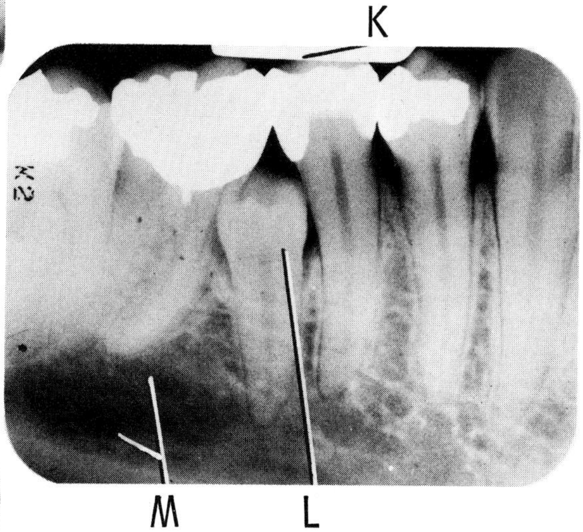

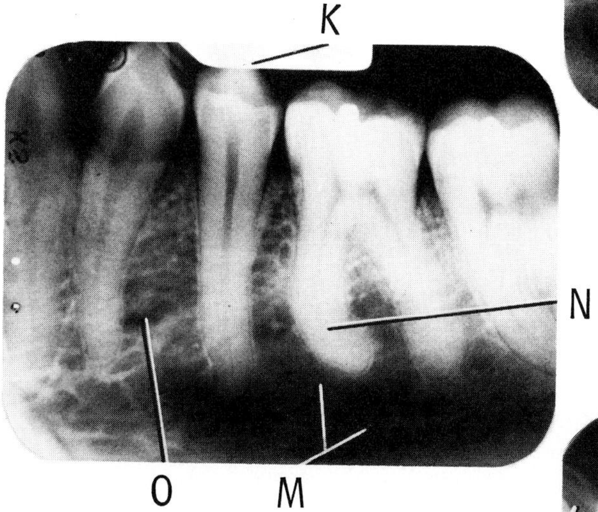

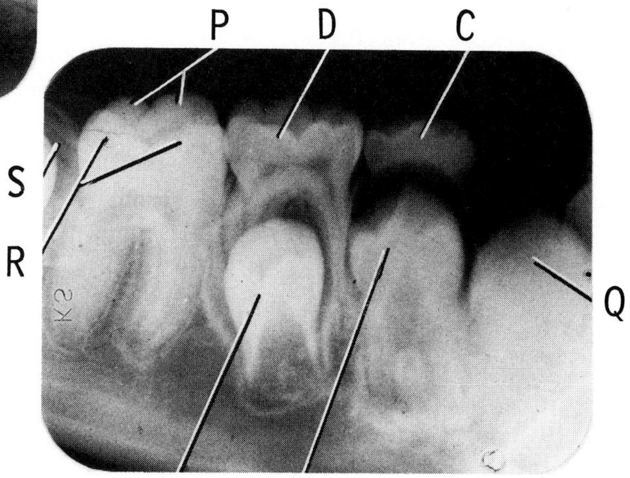

Plate 31   MANDIBULAR BICUSPID REGION VIEW _____

A.   Torn film emulsion
B.   Buccal cusp of mandibular permanent first bicuspid
C.   Lingual cusp of mandibular permanent first bicuspid
D.   Portion of metal film holder
E.   Metal restorations
F.   Submandibular fossa
G.   Internal oblique ridge
H.   Mandibular canal
I.   Mental foramen
J.   Sclerotic bone
K.   Film identification dot
L.   Shadow of portion of wooden film holder
M.   Resorbed edentulous ridge
N.   Bent corner of film
O.   Cortical bone of inferior border of mandible
P.   Bifid root of mandibular permanent second bicuspid
Q.   Hypercementosed distal root—mandibular permanent first molar
R.   Mandibular primary cuspid
S.   Pulpally treated mandibular primary first molar
T.   Chrome steel crown
U.   Pulpally treated mandibular primary second molar
V.   Buccal cusps of mandibular first molar
W.   Partial view of unerupted mandibular permanent second molar
X.   Developing mandibular second bicuspid
Y.   Developing mandibular permanent first bicuspid
Z.   Developing mandibular permanent cuspid

Plate 31   MANDIBULAR BICUSPID REGION VIEW

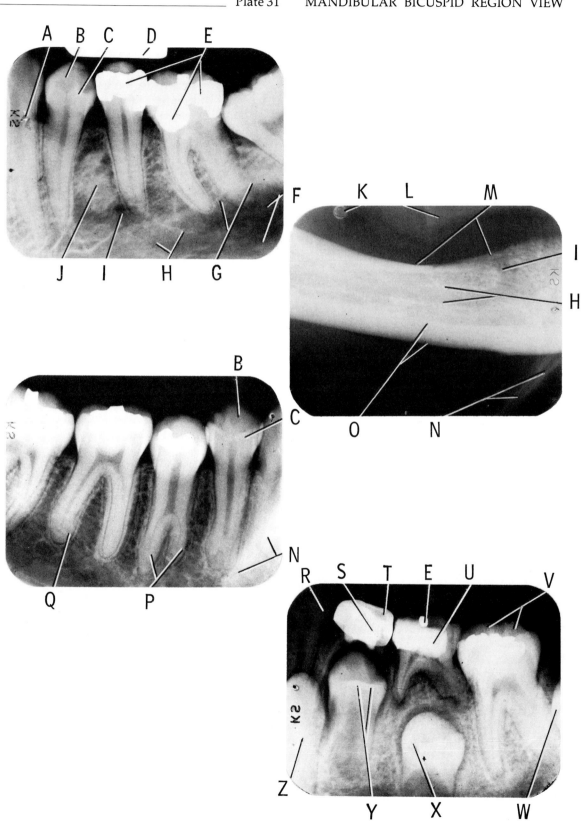

Plate 32   MANDIBULAR BICUSPID REGION VIEW ⎯⎯⎯⎯⎯⎯⎯⎯⎯⎯⎯⎯⎯⎯⎯⎯

A.   Supernumerary teeth
B.   Nutrient foramen

Plate 32   MANDIBULAR BICUSPID REGION VIEW

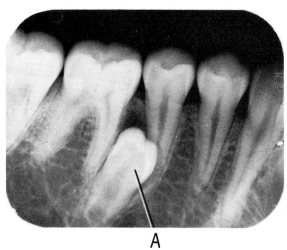

A

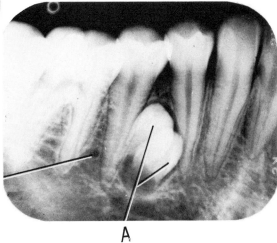

B

A

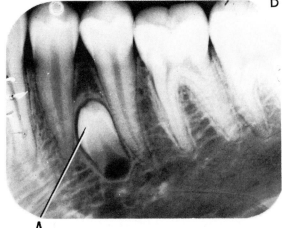

A

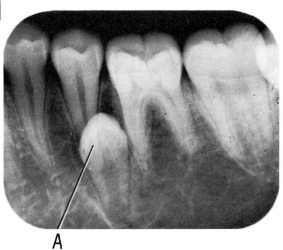

A

Plate 33   MANDIBULAR BICUSPID–MOLAR REGION VIEW _____

A.   Pulp canal recession due to indirect pulp capping procedure
B.   Cervical burnout (adumbration)
C.   Mental foramen
D.   Film crease
E.   Sclerotic bone (osteosclerosis)
F.   Mandibular canal
G.   Portion of impacted mandibular permanent third molar
H.   Carious lesions
I.   Condensing osteitis
J.   Radiolucency indicating pulpal pathology, probably due to operative
       pulp damage
K.   Periodontal interradicular radiolucency indicating bone resorption and
       pathology
L.   Radiolucency around crown of erupting mandibular permanent sec-
       ond bicuspid
M.   Developing root of mandibular permanent second bicuspid
N.   Submandibular fossa

Plate 33   MANDIBULAR BICUSPID–MOLAR REGION VIEW

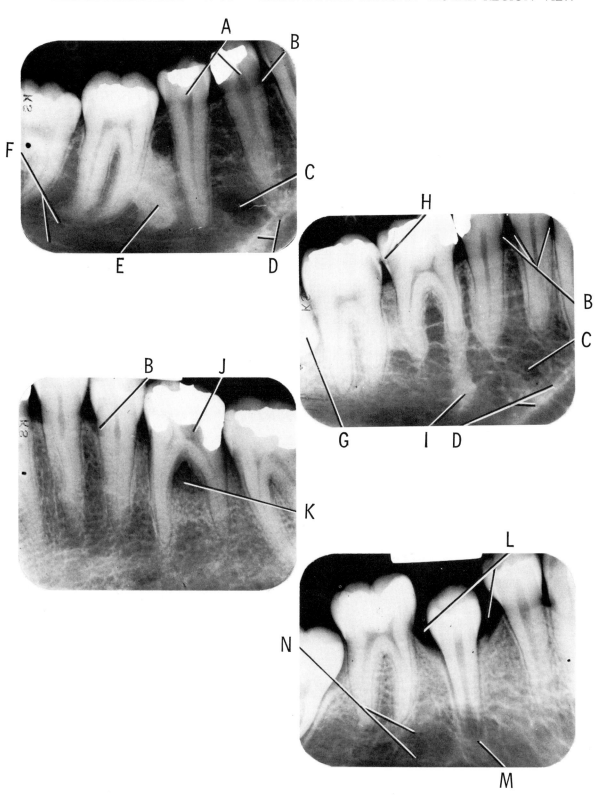

Plate 34   MANDIBULAR BICUSPID–MOLAR REGION VIEW _____

A.   Internal oblique ridge
B.   External oblique ridge
C.   Film identification dot
D.   Mandibular canal
E.   Dilacerated roots
F.   Portion of metal film holder
G.   Remnant of primary second molar
H.   Area of resorbed bone over erupting permanent second molar
I.   Follicle of developing permanent second bicuspid
J.   Caries
K.   Submandibular fossa

Plate 34   MANDIBULAR BICUSPID–MOLAR REGION VIEW

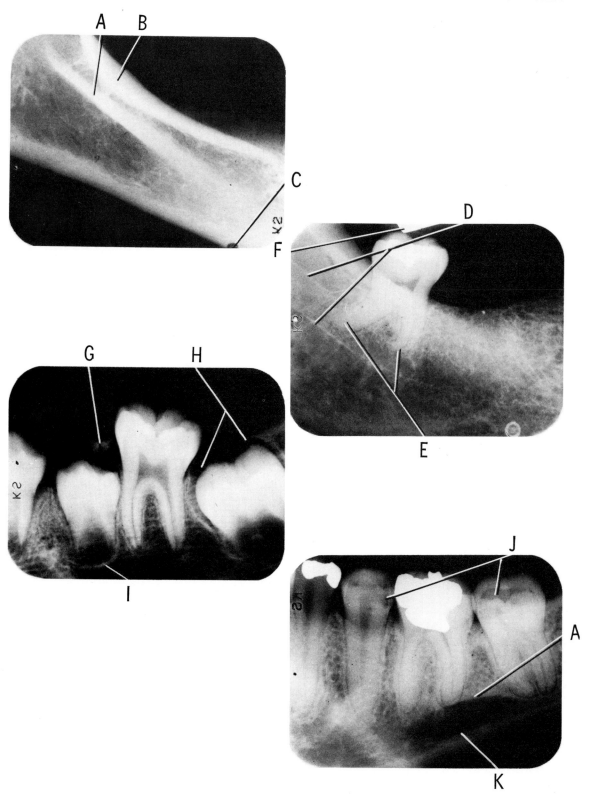

Plate 35   MANDIBULAR BICUSPID–MOLAR REGION VIEW _____

A.   Submandibular fossa
B.   Ankylosed mandibular primary second molar with no developing permanent second bicuspid
C.   Alveolar bone level
D.   Film identification dot
E.   Lingual cusp of mandibular permanent first bicuspid
F.   Buccal cusp of mandibular permanent first bicuspid
G.   Impacted mandibular permanent second bicuspid
H.   Chrome steel band and loop space maintainer
I.   Metal portion of film holder
J.   Crown of developing mandibular permanent second bicuspid
K.   Crown of developing mandibular permanent first bicuspid
L.   Retained remnant of primary molar root

Plate 35   MANDIBULAR BICUSPID–MOLAR REGION VIEW

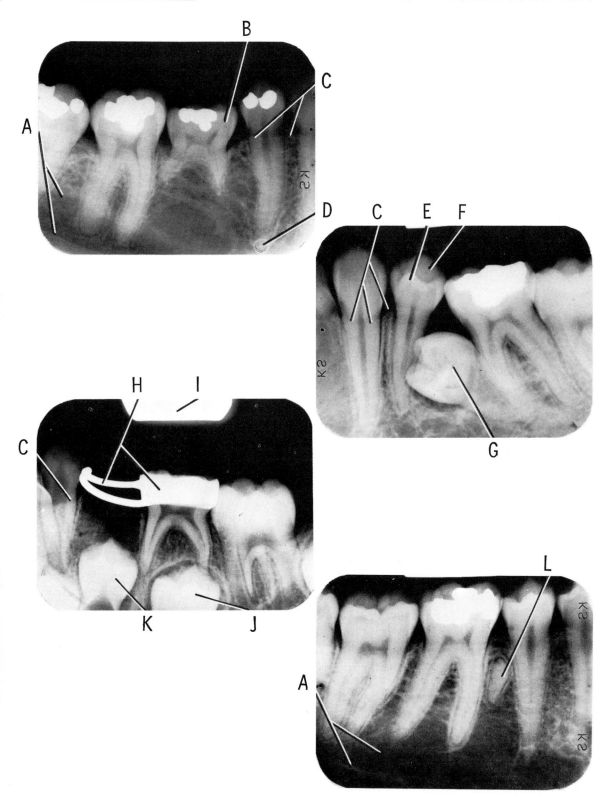

Plate 36   MANDIBULAR BICUSPID–MOLAR REGION VIEW _____

A.   Film crease
B.   Mental foramen
C.   Cortical bone of inferior border of mandible
D.   Overhanging metal restorations
E.   Mandibular canal
F.   Extraction site of mandibular molar
G.   Extraction site of mandibular bicuspid
H.   Lamina dura
I.   Retained root tip in soft tissue
J.   Large carious lesion

Plate 36   MANDIBULAR BICUSPID–MOLAR REGION VIEW

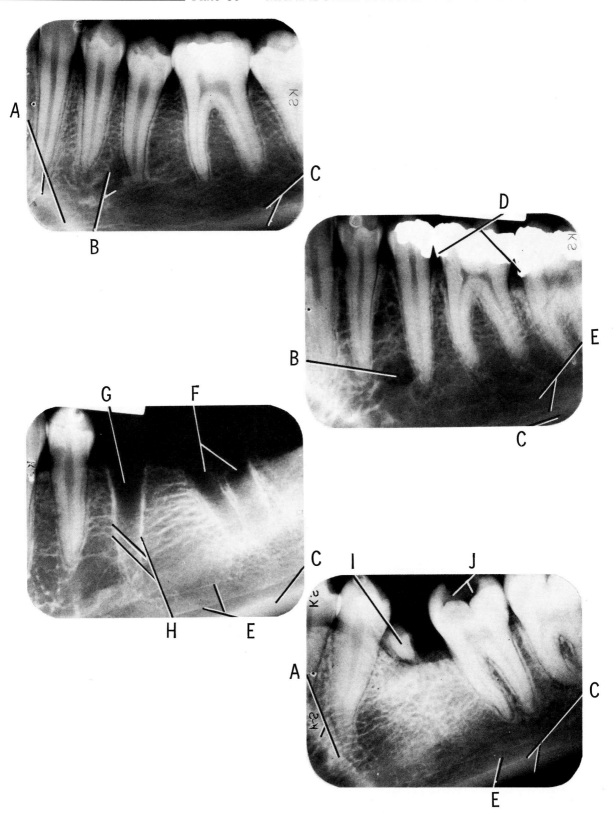

Plate 37   MANDIBULAR CUSPID REGION VIEW _____

A.   Enamel hypoplasia
B.   Internal oblique ridge
C.   Submandibular fossa
D.   Cortical plate of inferior border of mandible
E.   Mandibular primary lateral incisor
F.   Mandibular primary cuspid
G.   Mandibular primary first molar
H.   Mandibular primary second molar
I.   Mandibular permanent first bicuspid
J.   Mandibular permanent second bicuspid
K.   Mandibular permanent cuspid
L.   Mandibular permanent lateral incisor

Plate 37   MANDIBULAR CUSPID REGION VIEW

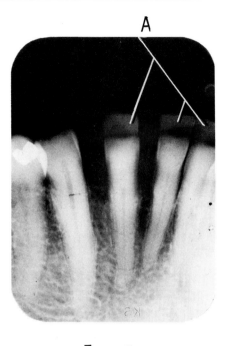

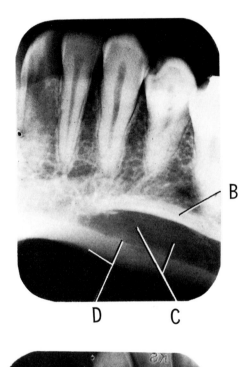

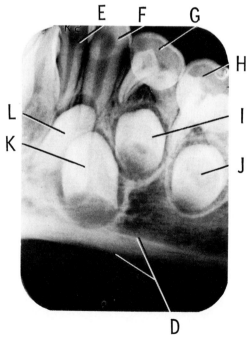

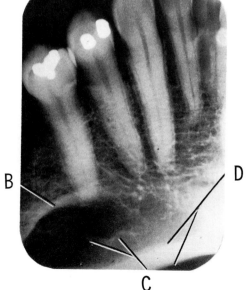

Plate 38   MANDIBULAR CUSPID REGION VIEW

A.   Lip line
B.   Area of bone loss
C.   Alveolar bone ridge line
D.   Cervical abrasion
E.   Sclerotic bone
F.   Calculus
G.   Metal film holder
H.   Genial tubercle
I.   Lingual foramen
J.   Impacted mandibular permanent cuspid

Plate 38   MANDIBULAR CUSPID REGION VIEW

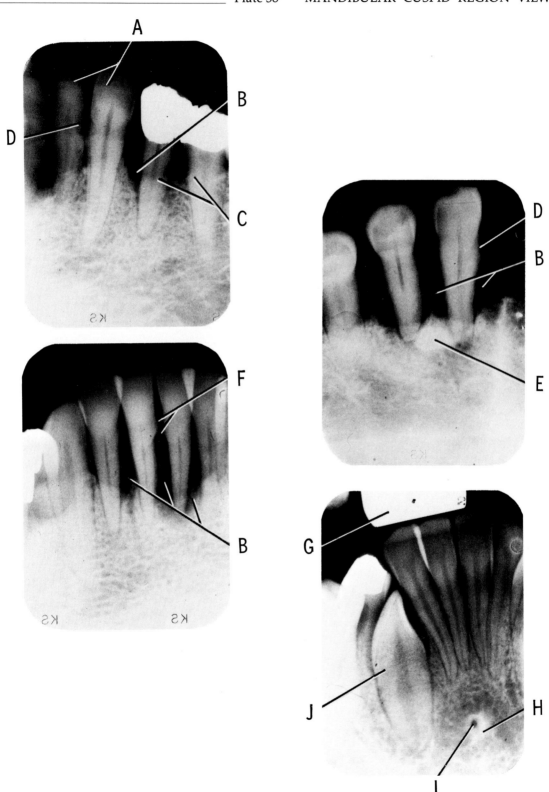

Plate 39   MANDIBULAR CUSPID REGION VIEW _____

A.   Cervical burnout (adumbration)
B.   Shadow of alveolar bone level
C.   Calculus
D.   Area of bone resorption
E.   Developing mandibular permanent cuspid
F.   Exfoliating mandibular primary molar
G.   Developing root of mandibular permanent cuspid
H.   Cortical bone of inferior border of mandible
I.   Shadow of wooden film holder
J.   Superimposition of mandibular permanent first bicuspid over permanent cuspid

Plate 39   MANDIBULAR CUSPID REGION VIEW

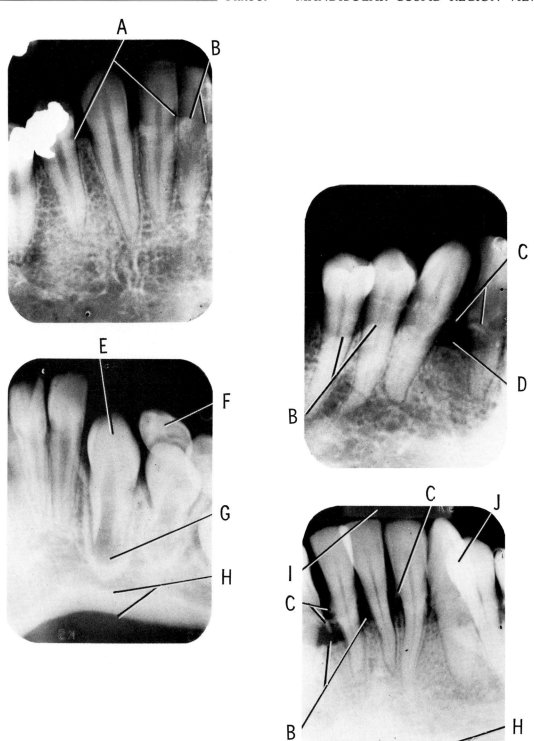

Plate 40   MANDIBULAR CUSPID REGION VIEW _____

A.   Unerupted mandibular permanent cuspid in follicle
B.   Mandibular primary first molar
C.   Mandibular primary cuspid — root resorbed
D.   Cortical bone of inferior border of mandible
E.   Recurrent caries
F.   Periapical radiolucency due to large carious lesions
G.   Alveolar bone level
H.   Normal trabecular bone pattern
I.   Occlusal and incisal abrasion
J.   Fixer chemical stain

Plate 40   MANDIBULAR CUSPID REGION VIEW

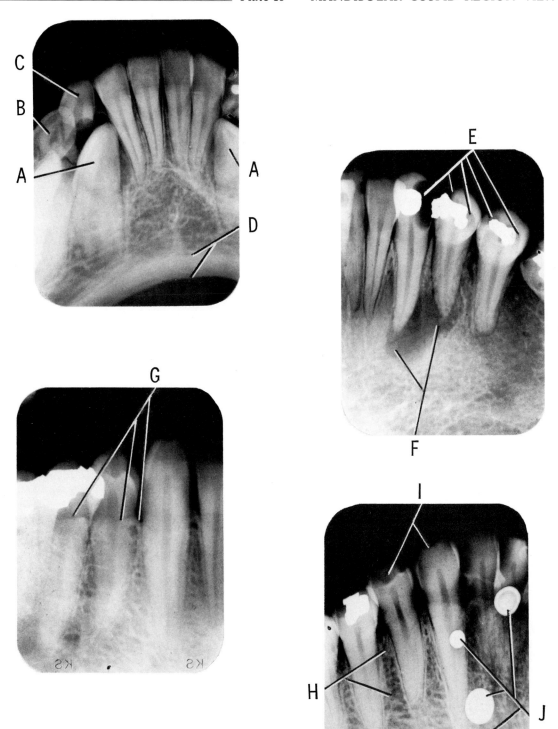

Plate 41   MANDIBULAR INCISOR REGION VIEW

A.   Fractured enamel
B.   Overlapped contacts
C.   Abrasion
D.   Level of alveolar bone
E.   Lingual foramen
F.   Lip line
G.   Genial tubercle
H.   Film crease
I.   Cortical bone – inferior border of mandible
J.   Narrow pulp canal (due to attrition)
K.   Sclerosed pulp chamber (due to attrition)
L.   Attrition
M.   Mamelons
N.   Film identification dot
O.   Radiolucency of follicle around unerupted permanent cuspid

Plate 41   MANDIBULAR INCISOR REGION VIEW

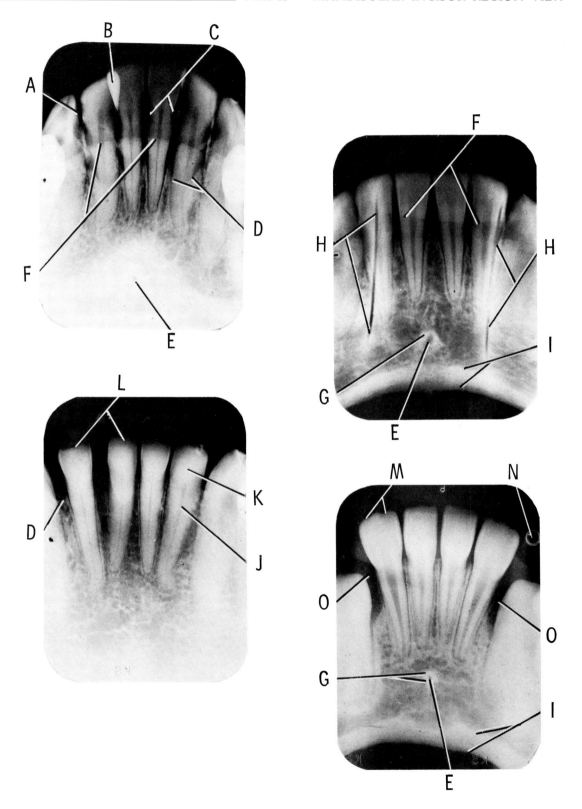

Plate 42   MANDIBULAR INCISOR REGION VIEW _____

A.   Radiolucent resin restorations
B.   Normal thin bone
C.   Genial tubercle
D.   Incisal abrasion
E.   Radiopaque calculus bridge
F.   Alveolar ridge bone line
G.   Nutrient foramen
H.   Nutrient canals
I.   Lip line
J.   Mental ridge
K.   Unerupted mandibular permanent cuspid
L.   Cortical bone of inferior border of mandible
M.   Gold crown restoration of mandibular permanent cuspid

Plate 42   MANDIBULAR INCISOR REGION VIEW

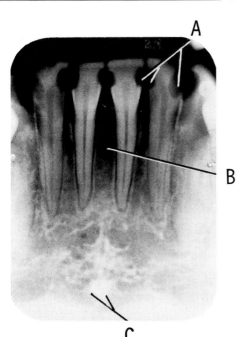

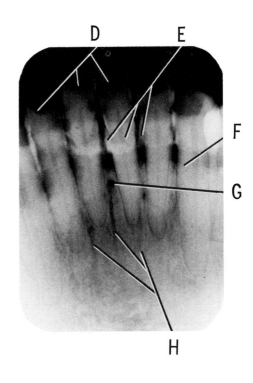

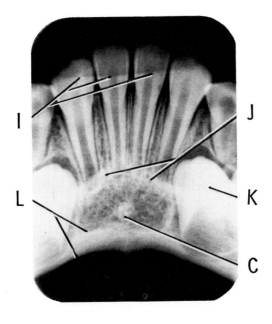

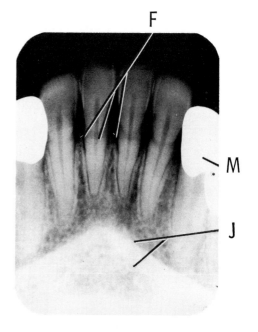

Plate 43   MANDIBULAR INCISOR REGION VIEW _____

A.   Permanent lateral incisor
B.   Permanent central incisor
C.   Overlapping contacts
D.   Permanent cuspid
E.   Genial tubercle
F.   Lingual foramen
G.   Inferior cortical plate of border of mandible
H.   Enamel
I.   Shadow of lip
J.   Calculus
K.   Alveolar bone ridge
L.   Metal film holder
M.   Rubber material surrounding film holder
N.   Film identification dot
O.   Line of fracture
P.   Metal wire used to repair fracture
Q.   Developing permanent lateral incisors in follicles
R.   Permanent central incisors with incompletely developed roots
S.   Primary lateral incisor
T.   Primary cuspid

Plate 43   MANDIBULAR INCISOR REGION VIEW

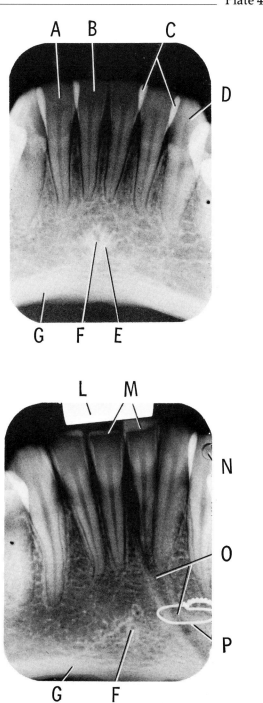

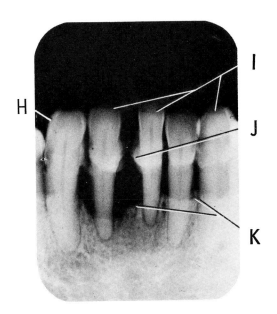

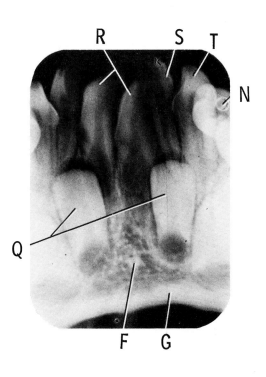

Plate 44   BITEWING VIEW OF BICUSPID–MOLAR REGION _____

A. External oblique ridge
B. Overcontoured gold crown restoration
C. Healed extraction site
D. Fractured area of crown
E. Maxillary full denture prosthetic teeth
F. Metal pin on lingual side of prosthetic cuspid tooth
G. Radiolucent space between gold restoration and tooth preparation
H. Endodontic filling material
I. Portion of mandibular permanent molar
J. Pulp stones
K. Cervical burnout (adumbration)
L. Maxillary tuberosity

Plate 44   BITEWING VIEW OF BICUSPID–MOLAR REGION

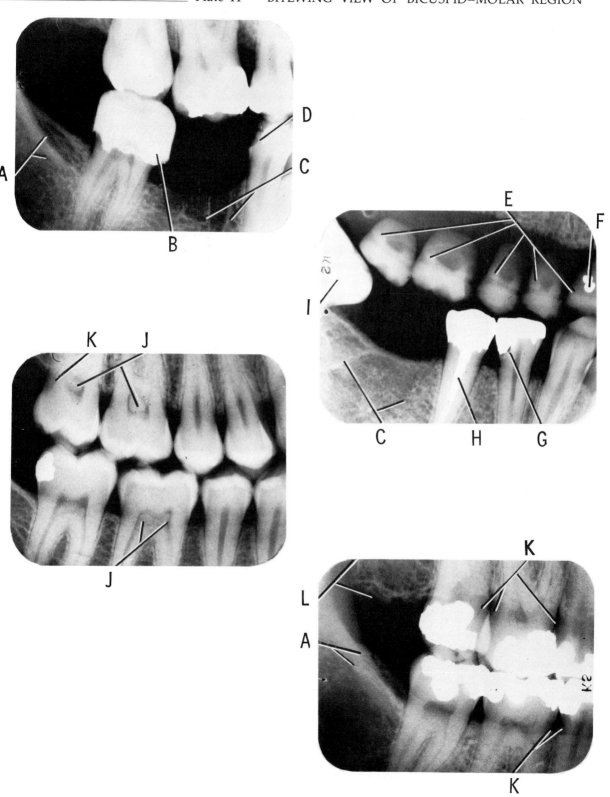

Plate 45   BITEWING VIEW OF BICUSPID–MOLAR REGION _____

A.   Endodontic restoration material
B.   Overhanging restoration
C.   Gold crown restoration
D.   Bone level
E.   Metal reinforcing pins under gold crown restoration are not in pulp
          chamber
F.   Floor of the maxillary sinus
G.   External oblique ridge of mandible
H.   Cervical burnout (adumbration)
I.   Film identification dot
J.   Portion of unerupted mandibular permanent third molar

Plate 45   BITEWING VIEW OF BICUSPID–MOLAR REGION

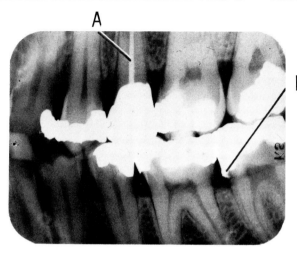

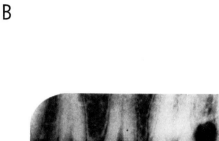

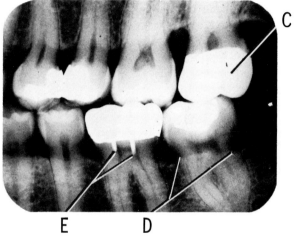

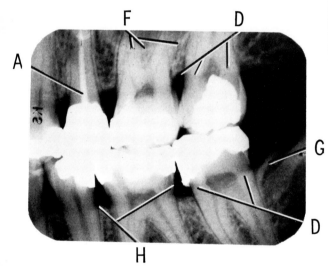

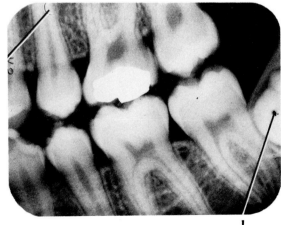

Plate 46   BITEWING VIEW OF BICUSPID–MOLAR REGION _____

A.	Pulp stone
B.	Cement base under silver alloy restoration
C.	Silver alloy restoration in buccal pit
D.	Root canal
E.	Enamel
F.	Pulp chamber
G.	Carious lesion

Plate 46   BITEWING VIEW OF BICUSPID–MOLAR REGION

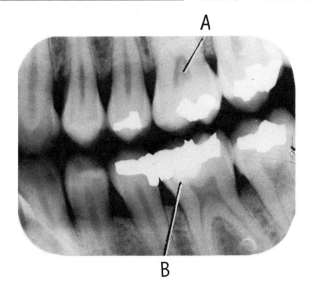

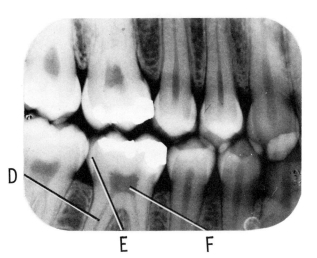

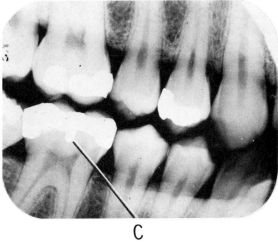

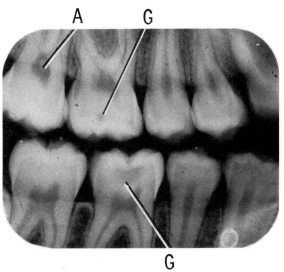

Plate 47   BITEWING VIEW OF BICUSPID–MOLAR REGION

A.   Poorly contoured silver alloy restoration
B.   Carious lesion
C.   Recurrent carious lesion
D.   Pulp stone
E.   Cement base under silver alloy restoration
F.   Secondary dentin
G.   Level of alveolar bone
H.   Erupting maxillary permanent second bicuspid
I.   Crown remnant of maxillary primary second molar

Plate 47   BITEWING VIEW OF BICUSPID–MOLAR REGION

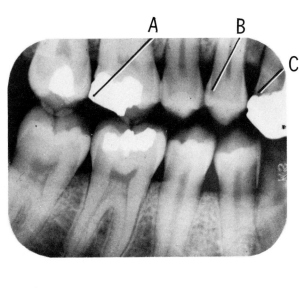

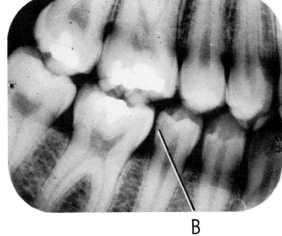

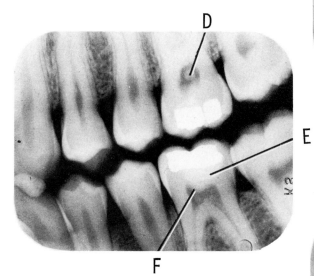

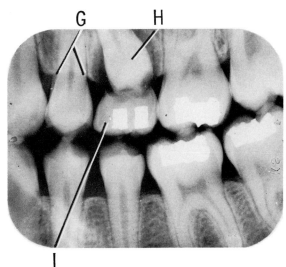

Plate 48   MAXILLARY ANTERIOR OCCLUSAL VIEW _____

A.   Nasal septum
B.   Nasal fossa
C.   Anterior nasal spine
D.   Nasal concha
E.   Impacted permanent central incisor
F.   Cone cut
G.   Fractured crown, permanent lateral incisor
H.   Periapical radiolucency
I.   Incisive foramen
J.   Median palatal suture
K.   Maxillary sinus
L.   Zygomatic process of maxilla

Plate 48   MAXILLARY ANTERIOR OCCLUSAL VIEW

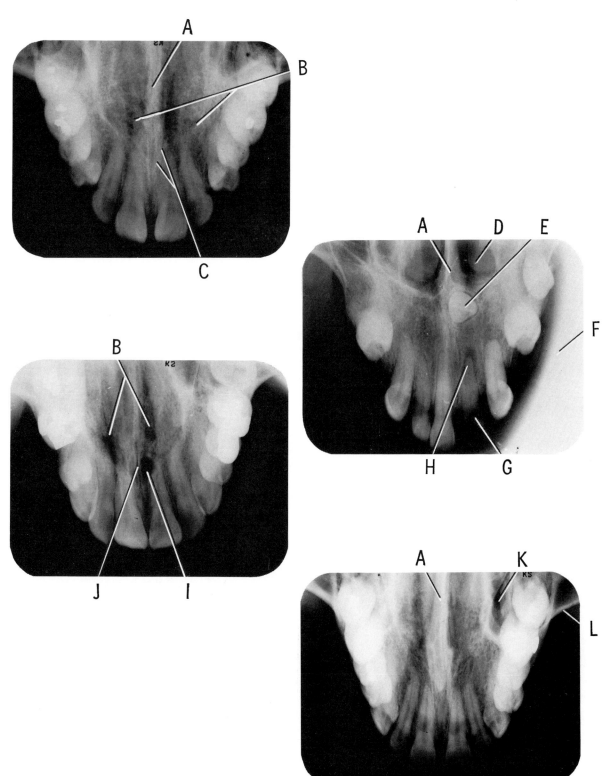

Plate 49   MAXILLARY ANTERIOR OCCLUSAL VIEW _____

A. Nasal fossa
B. Nasal septum
C. Median palatal suture
D. Maxillary sinus
E. Anterior nasal spine
F. Root canal filling
G. Jacket crown preparation
H. Superior foramina of incisive canal
I. Cone cut
J. Gold crown restorations
K. Zygomatic process of maxilla
L. Lateral border of nasal fossa
M. Cartilaginous septum of nose
N. Nasolacrimal duct
O. Porcelain denture teeth with metal pins
P. Retained root
Q. Retained impacted tooth

Plate 49   MAXILLARY ANTERIOR OCCLUSAL VIEW

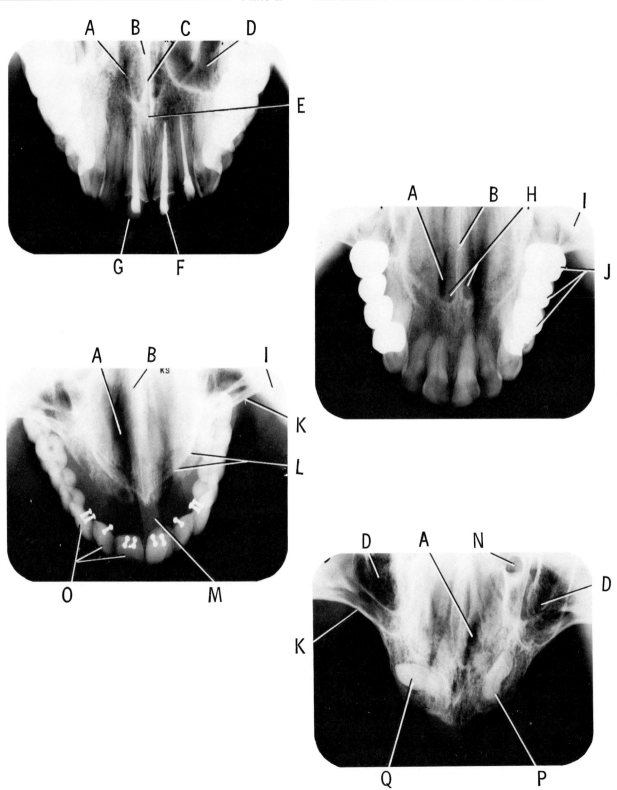

Plate 50   MANDIBULAR ANTERIOR OCCLUSAL VIEW _____

A.   Mental ridge
B.   Genial tubercle
C.   External oblique ridge
D.   Shadow of tongue
E.   Cone cut

Plate 50   MANDIBULAR ANTERIOR OCCLUSAL VIEW

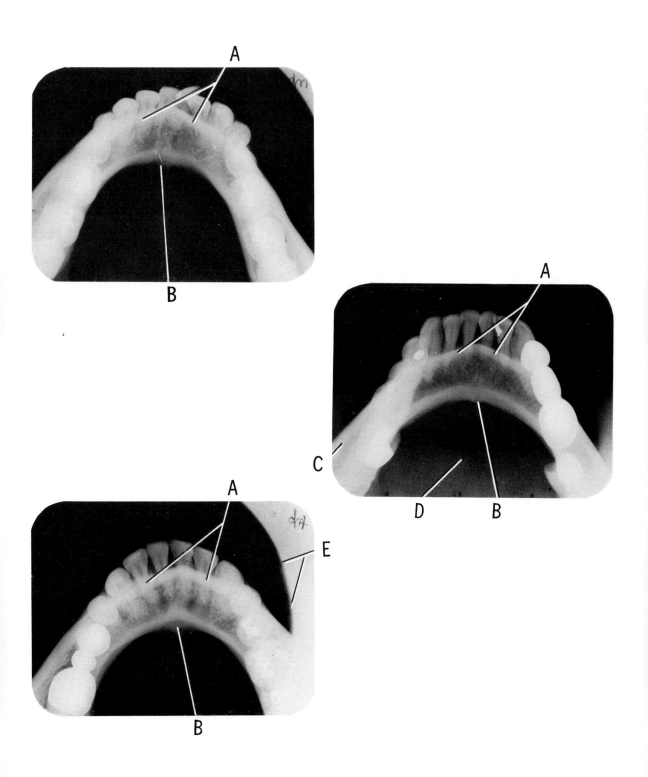

section two

EXTRAORAL RADIOGRAPHS OF THE HUMAN SKULL

Plate 51   LATERAL OBLIQUE JAW VIEW _____

A. Shadow of spinal vertebrae
B. Zygomatic arch
C. Coronoid process of mandible
D. Shadow of the tongue
E. Inferior border of opposite side of mandible
F. Mental foramen
G. Mandibular canal
H. Hyoid bone
I. Maxillary arch
J. Wire used to repair earlier fracture
K. Posterior wall of pharynx
L. Mandibular condyle

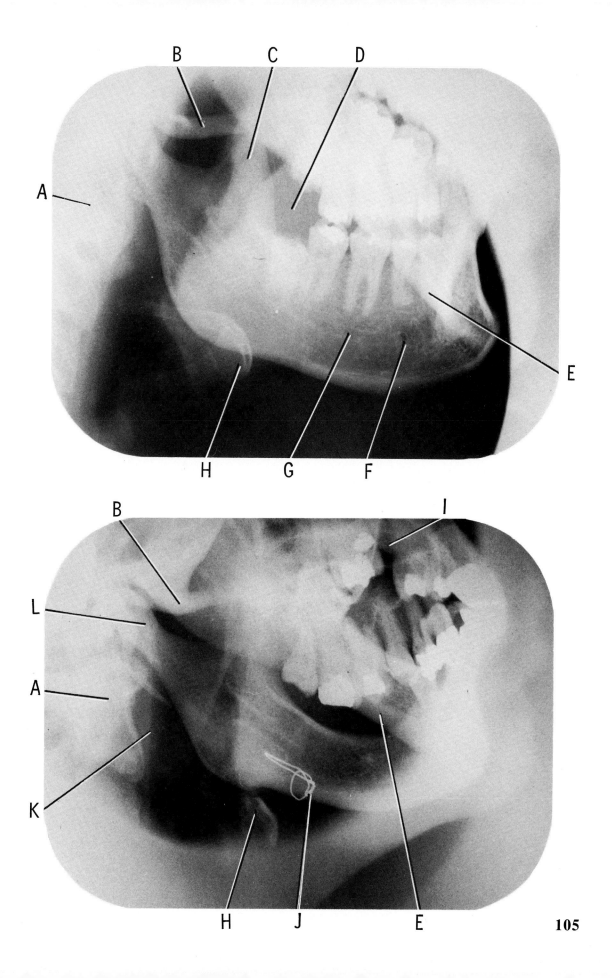

Plate 52   LATERAL OBLIQUE JAW VIEW _____

A.   Maxillary sinus
B.   Inferior border of opposite side of mandible
C.   Mental foramen
D.   Hyoid bone
E.   Cortical bone of inferior border of mandible
F.   Shadow of spinal vertebrae
G.   External oblique ridge
H.   Mandibular canal
I.   Mandibular foramen
J.   Sigmoid notch
K.   Coronoid process
L.   Zygomatic arch

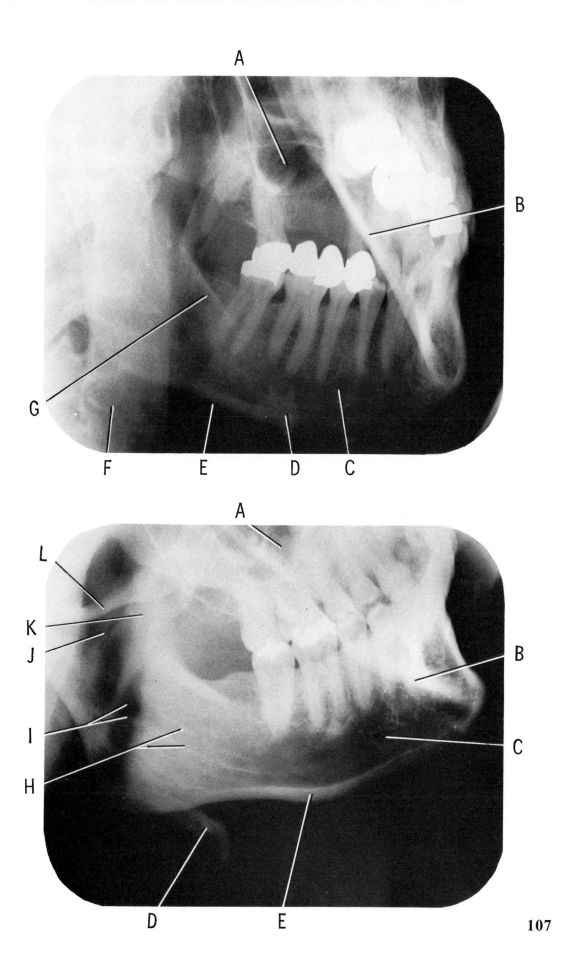

Plate 53   LATERAL OBLIQUE JAW VIEW _____

A.   Oropharynx
B.   Shadow of tongue
C.   Porcelain teeth of maxillary denture
D.   Mental foramen
E.   Mandibular canal
F.   Mandibular condyle
G.   Articular eminence
H.   Zygomatic arch
I.   Coronoid process of mandible
J.   Facial artery notch
K.   Styloid process

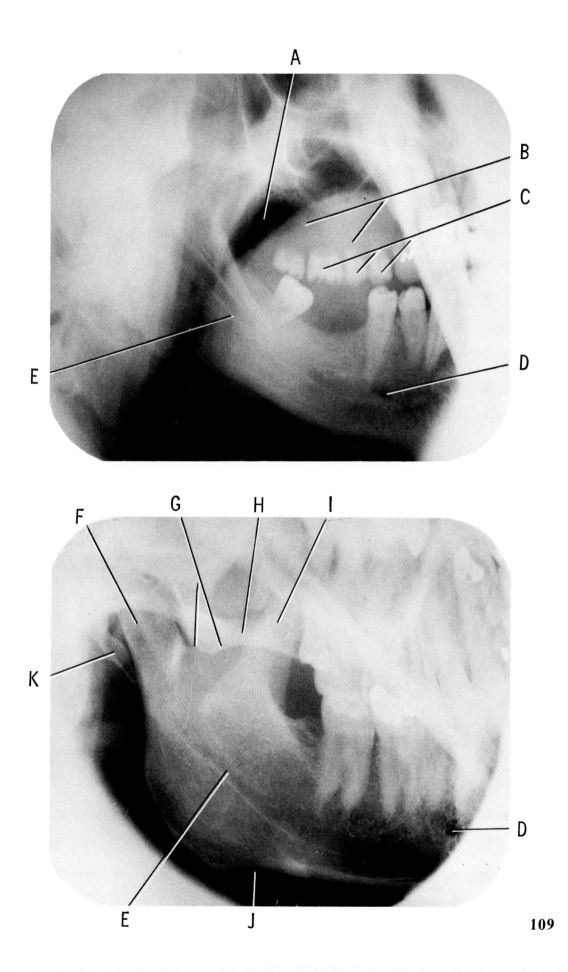

Plate 54   LATERAL OBLIQUE JAW VIEW _____

A.   Zygomatic arch
B.   Shadow of soft tissue of face
C.   Inferior border of opposite side of mandible
D.   Mental foramen
E.   Mandibular canal
F.   External oblique ridge
G.   Wall of pharynx
H.   Styloid process

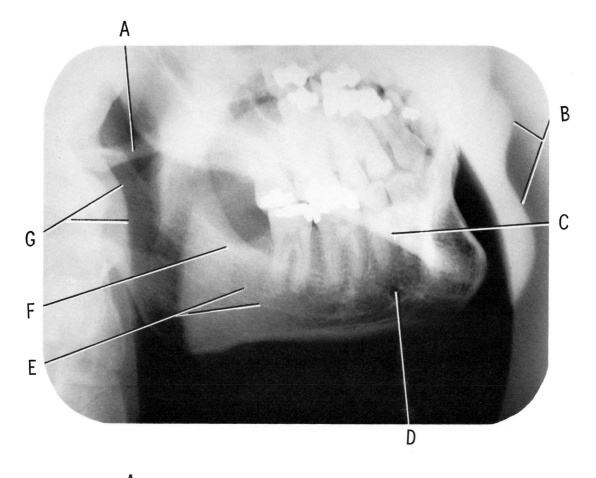

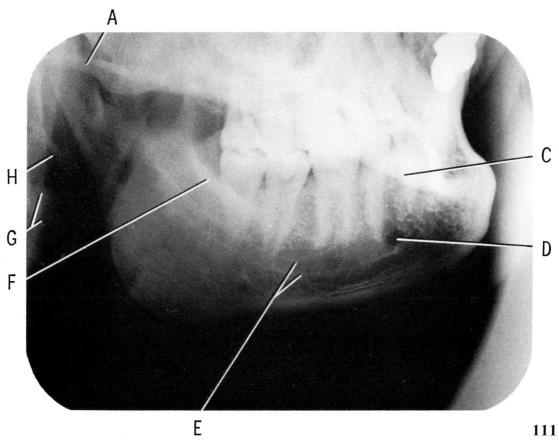

Plate 55   PANORAMIC VIEW ——————————————————————————————————

A. Maxillary tuberosity
B. Shadow of hard palate
C. Zygoma
D. Maxillary sinus
E. Coronoid process of mandible
F. Articular eminence
G. Glenoid fossa
H. Mandibular condyle
I. Styloid process
J. Mandibular canal
K. External oblique ridge
L. Metal bite-block
M. Shadow of tongue
N. Space between tongue and soft palate
O. Shadow of soft palate

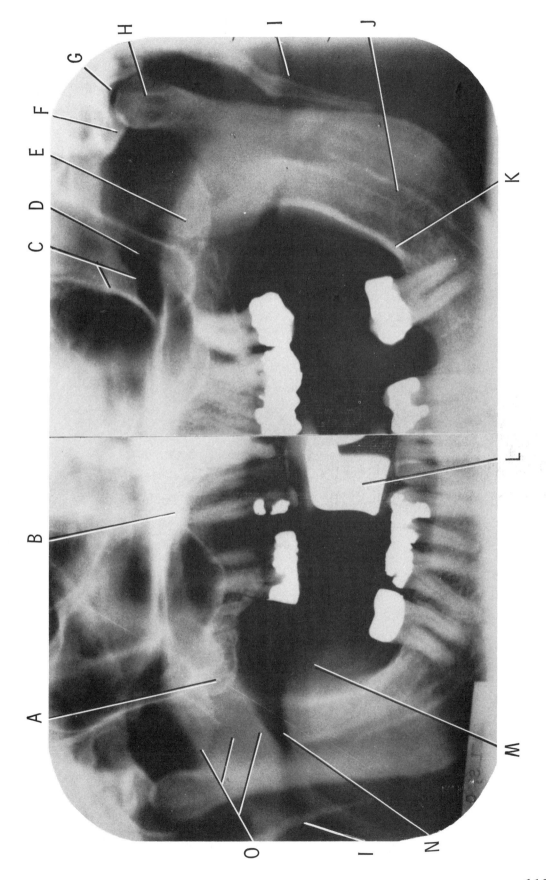

Plate 56   PANORAMIC VIEW (EDENTULOUS) _____

A.   Coronoid process of mandible
B.   Maxillary tuberosity
C.   Nasal fossa
D.   Nasal septum
E.   Hard palate
F.   Orbit
G.   Maxillary sinus
H.   Zygomatic arch
I.   Articular eminence
J.   Mandibular condyle
K.   Cervical vertebrae
L.   Facial artery notch
M.   Mandibular canal
N.   Plastic chin rest
O.   Symphysis
P.   Mental foramen
Q.   Shadow of tongue
R.   Angle of mandible
S.   Pharynx
T.   Mandibular foramen

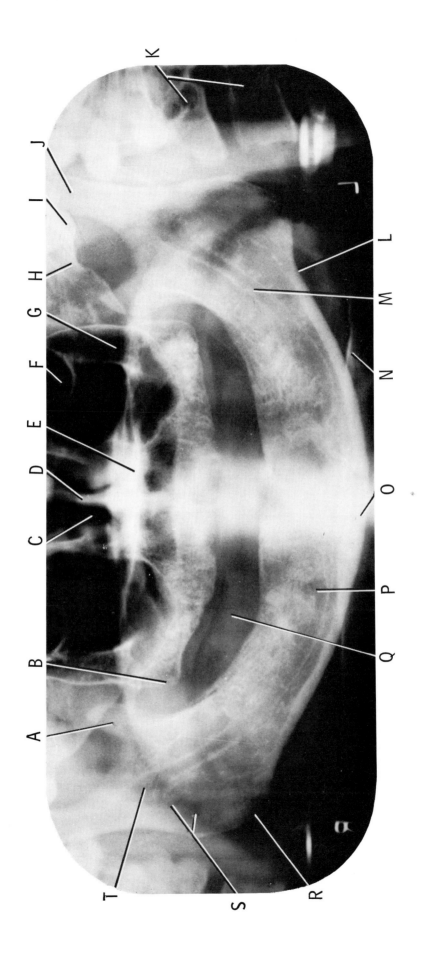

Plate 57   PANORAMIC VIEW (CHERUBISM) _____

A. Articular eminence
B. Coronoid process of mandible
C. Nasal concha
D. Nasal septum
E. Nasal fossa
F. Maxillary sinus
G. Symphysis
H. Plastic chin rest
I. Fibro-osseous lesion
J. Angle of mandible
K. Soft tissue of external ear (lobule)
L. Cervical vertebra
M. Mandibular condyle
N. External auditory meatus
O. Glenoid fossa

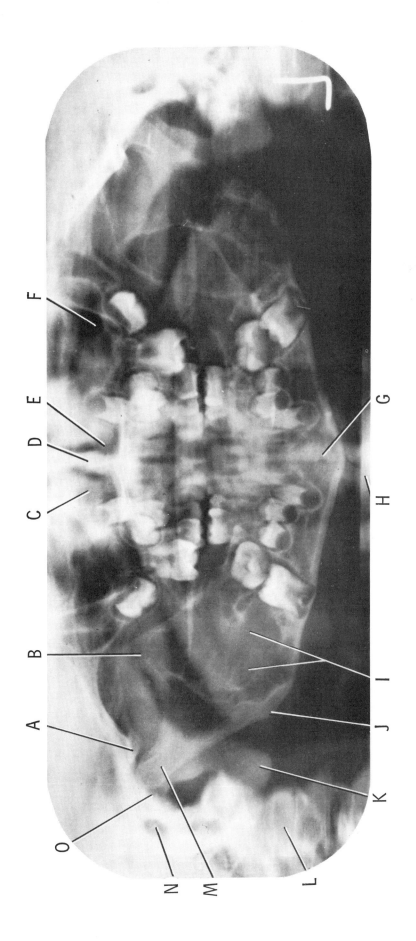

Plate 58   PANORAMIC VIEW _____

Film damaged by static electricity

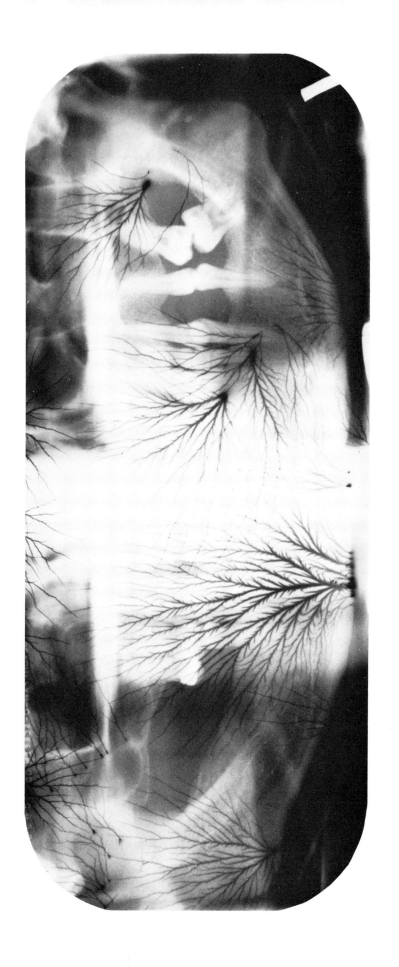

Plate 59   PANORAMIC VIEW _____

A. Nasal fossa
B. Nasal septum
C. Hard palate
D. Maxillary sinus
E. Zygomatic arch
F. Articular eminence
G. Glenoid fossa
H. Mandibular condyle
I. Mental foramen
J. Symphysis
K. Mandibular canal
L. Cervical vertebra
M. Mandibular foramen
N. Styloid process

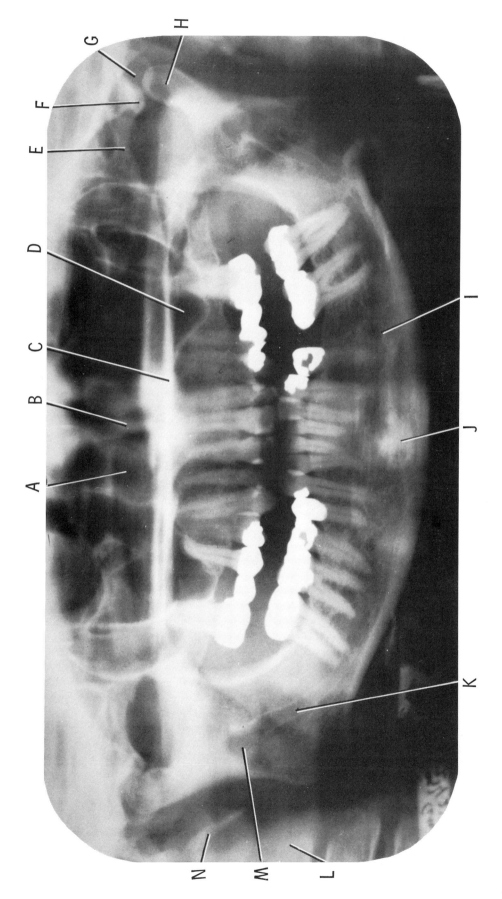

Plate 60   PANORAMIC VIEW

A. Maxillary sinus
B. Nasal fossa
C. Hard palate
D. Zygomatic arch
E. Mandibular canal
F. Oropharynx
G. Symphysis
H. External oblique ridge
I. Soft palate

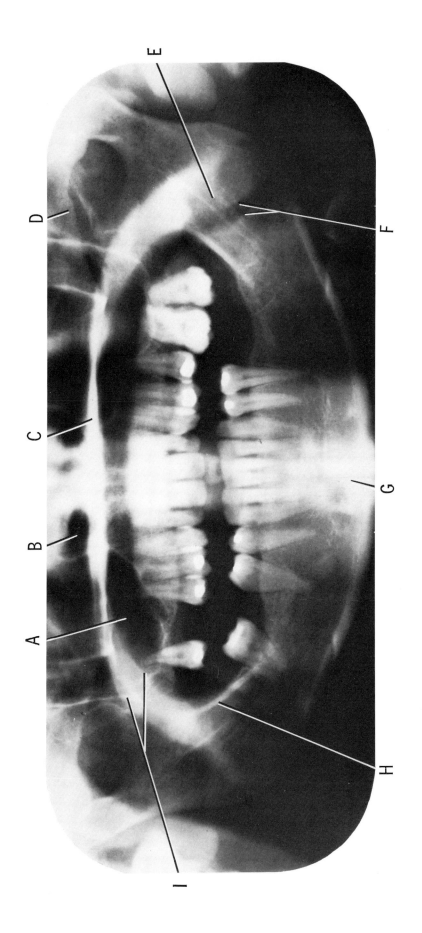

Plate 61   PANORAMIC VIEW (EDENTULOUS) _____

A. Mandibular notch
B. Nasal concha
C. Nasal septum
D. Nasal fossa
E. Hard palate
F. Articular eminence
G. Glenoid fossa
H. Mandibular condyle
I. External oblique ridge
J. Mental foramen
K. Shadow of ramus of opposite side

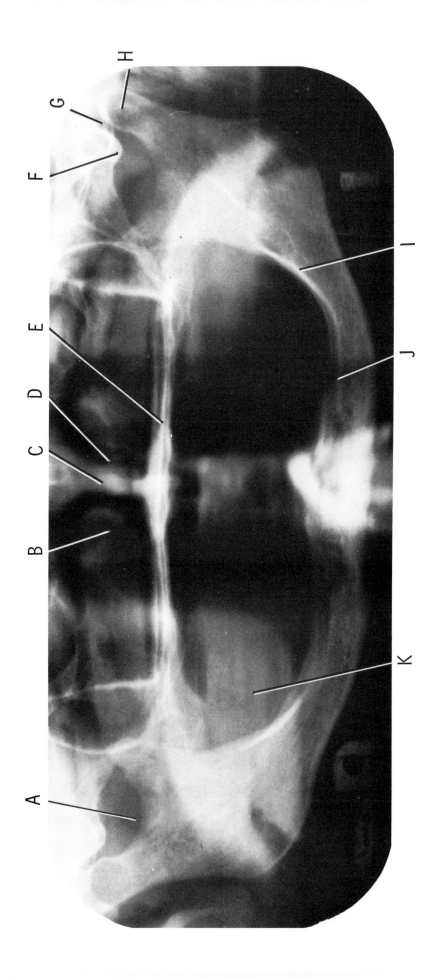

Plate 62   PANORAMIC VIEW

A. Maxillary sinus
B. Area of no radiation exposure
C. Nasal septum
D. Nasal fossa and concha
E. Hard palate
F. Plastic chin rest
G. Large carious lesion
H. Maxillary permanent lateral incisor
I. Maxillary permanent central incisor of opposite side
J. Carious lesion
K. Shadow of plastic chin rest of opposite side
L. Shadow of ramus of opposite side
M. Soft tissue of external ear (lobule)
N. External auditory meatus

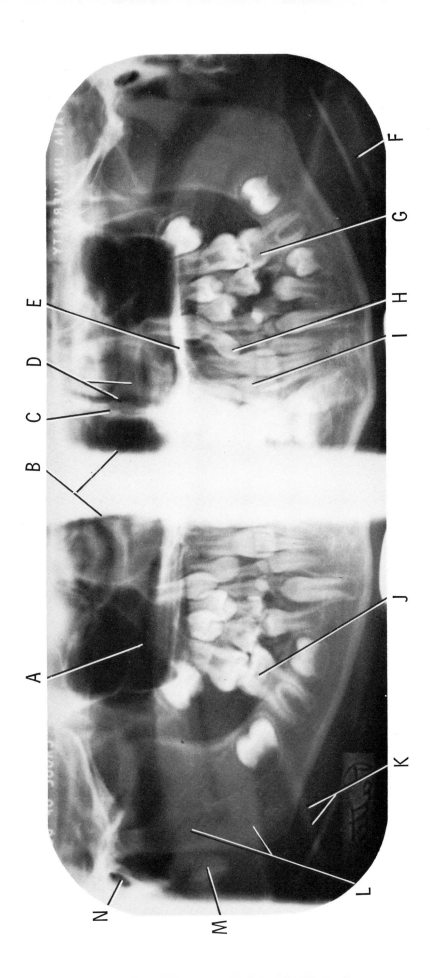

Plate 63   LATERAL HEADPLATE VIEW

A.   External cortical plate
B.   Internal cortical plate
C.   Coronal suture
D.   Artifact
E.   Anterior clinoid process
F.   Roof of orbit
G.   Nasal fossa
H.   Nasal bone
I.   Anterior nasal spine
J.   Developing mandibular permanent second molar in follicle
K.   Sphenoid sinus
L.   External auditory meatus
M.   Pituitary fossa in sella turcica
N.   Mastoid process
O.   Occipitomastoid suture
P.   Posterior clinoid process
Q.   Lambdoid suture
R.   Squamous suture

129

Plate 63   LATERAL HEADPLATE VIEW

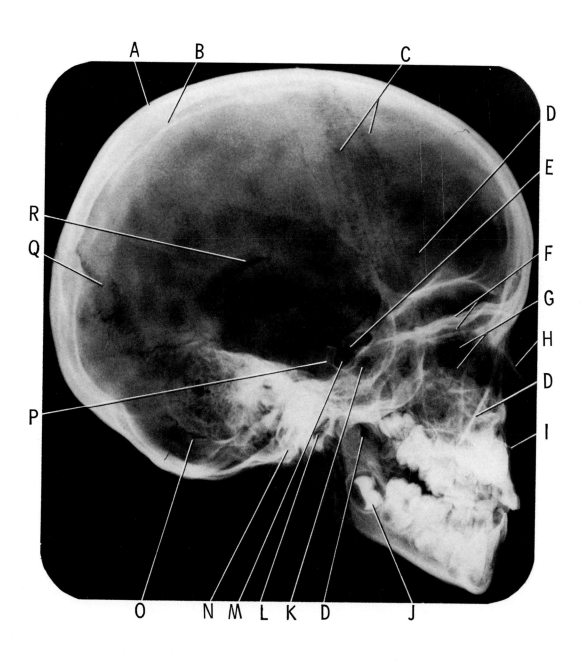

Plate 64   LATERAL HEADPLATE VIEW

A. Metal ear rod
B. Pituitary fossa in sella turcica
C. Roof of orbit
D. Anterior clinoid process
E. Frontal sinus
F. Plastic orbital pointer
G. Posterior clinoid process
H. Sphenoid sinus
I. Orbit
J. Nasal fossa
K. Anterior nasal spine
L. Floor of nasal fossa
M. Roof of maxillary sinus
N. Maxillary sinus

O. Posterior border of tongue
P. Oropharynx
Q. Hyoid bone
R. Posterior pharyngeal wall
S. Body of third cervical vertebra
T. Body of fourth cervical vertebra
U. Body of fifth cervical vertebra
V. Body of axis
W. Spinous processes of third, fourth and fifth cervical vertebrae
X. Soft palate
Y. Spinous process of axis
Z. Spinous process of atlas

a. Nasopharynx
b. Odontoid process of axis
c. Anterior tubercle of atlas
d. Occipital eminence

e. Occipital condyle
f. Mastoid air cells
g. Shadow of petrosal pyramid of temporal bone

Plate 64   LATERAL HEADPLATE VIEW

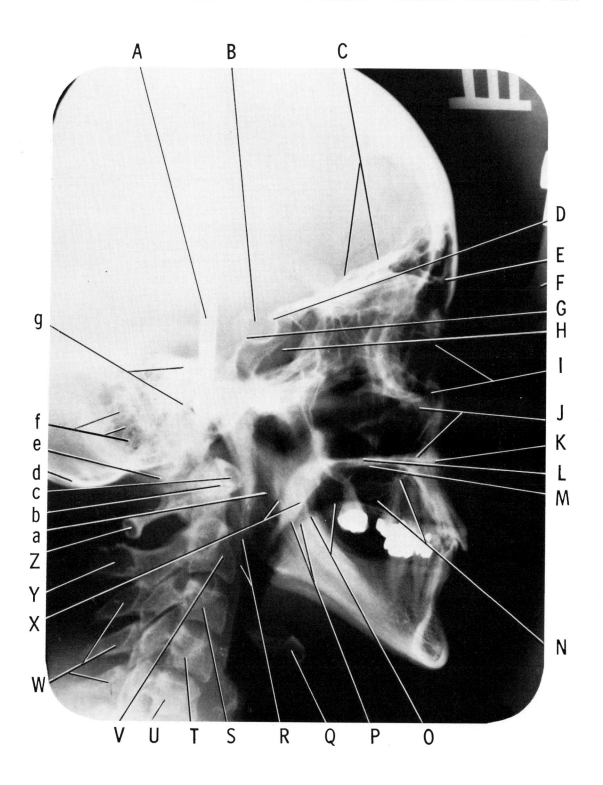

Plate 65   LATERAL HEADPLATE VIEW _____

A. Coronal suture
B. Inner cortical plate
C. Outer cortical plate
D. Roof of orbit
E. Frontal sinus
F. Orbit
G. Sphenoid sinus
H. Maxillary sinus superimposed over nasal fossa
I. Radiopaque material painted on the dorsum of the tongue
J. Lip of maxilla
K. Lip of mandible
L. Mandibular permanent first and second bicuspids
M. Mandibular permanent first and second molars

N. Unerupted mandibular permanent third molar
O. Soft palate
P. Hyoid bone
Q. Oropharynx
R. Nasopharynx
S. Fourth cervical vertebra
T. Third cervical vertebra
U. Axis
V. Atlas
W. Pituitary fossa in sella turcica
X. Mastoid air cells
Y. Plastic ear rod and head holder
Z. Posterior clinoid process

_____

a. Metal hairpins

Plate 65   LATERAL HEADPLATE VIEW

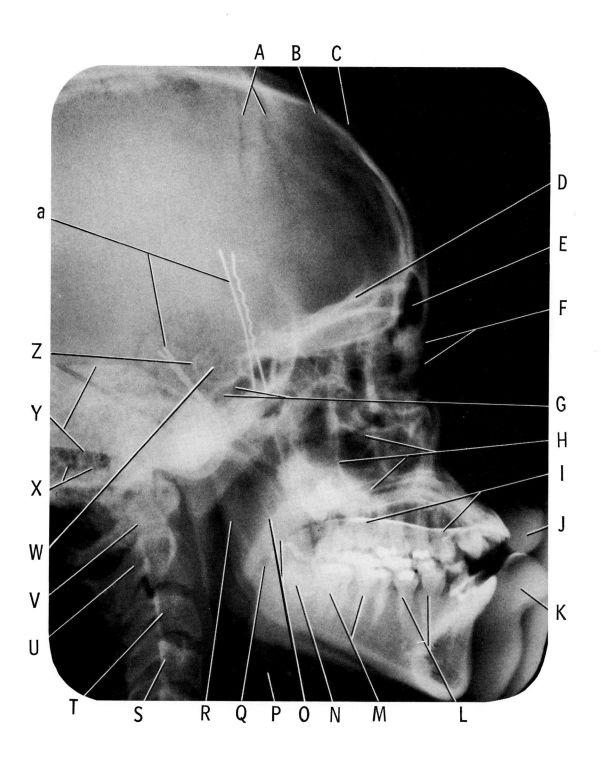

Plate 66   LATERAL HEADPLATE VIEW

A.   Patient identification plate
B.   Inner cortical plate
C.   Outer cortical plate
D.   Posterior clinoid process
E.   Pituitary fossa in sella turcica
F.   Roof of orbit
G.   Anterior clinoid process
H.   Frontal sinus
I.   Sphenoid sinus
J.   Orbit
K.   Maxillary sinus superimposed over nasal fossa
L.   Hard palate
M.   Unerupted maxillary permanent cuspid

N.   Maxillary permanent first bicuspid
O.   Maxillary permanent second bicuspid
P.   Maxillary permanent first molar
Q.   Maxillary primary molars
R.   Mandibular permanent first bicuspid
S.   Mandibular primary second molar
T.   Mandibular permanent second bicuspid
U.   Mandibular permanent first molar
V.   Maxillary permanent second molar
W.   Mandibular permanent second molar
X.   Hyoid bone
Y.   Oropharynx
Z.   Soft palate

a.   Nasopharynx
b.   Pharyngeal wall
c.   Fourth cervical vertebra
d.   Third cervical vertebra
e.   Axis
f.   Atlas

g.   Odontoid process of axis
h.   Mastoid air cells
i.   Outer cortical plate of occipital bone
j.   Inner cortical plate of occipital bone
k.   Plastic ear rod and head holder
l.   Lambdoid suture

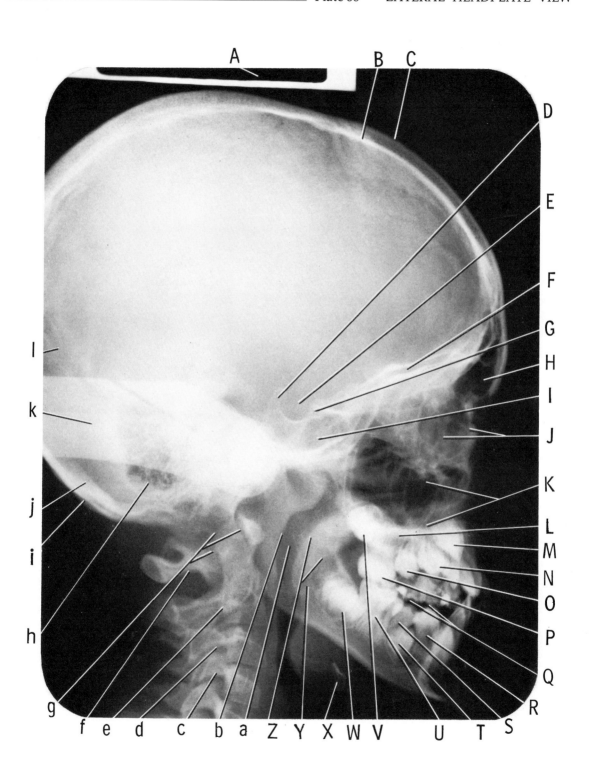

Plate 67   POSTEROANTERIOR HEADPLATE VIEW _____

A.   Sagittal suture
B.   Coronal suture
C.   Greater wing of sphenoid
D.   Superior border of orbit
E.   Nasal septum
F.   Nasal concha
G.   Primary central incisor of maxilla
H.   Unerupted permanent first molar of mandible
I.   Angle of mandible
J.   Inferior border of mandible
K.   Shadow of cervical vertebrae
L.   Primary cuspid of mandible
M.   Unerupted mandibular permanent central incisor
N.   Unerupted mandibular permanent lateral incisor
O.   Unerupted mandibular permanent cuspid
P.   Mandibular primary left central incisor
Q.   Mandibular primary right central incisor
R.   Unerupted maxillary permanent central incisor
S.   Unerupted maxillary permanent first molar
T.   Maxillary sinus
U.   Foramen rotundum
V.   Crista galli

Plate 67   POSTEROANTERIOR HEADPLATE VIEW

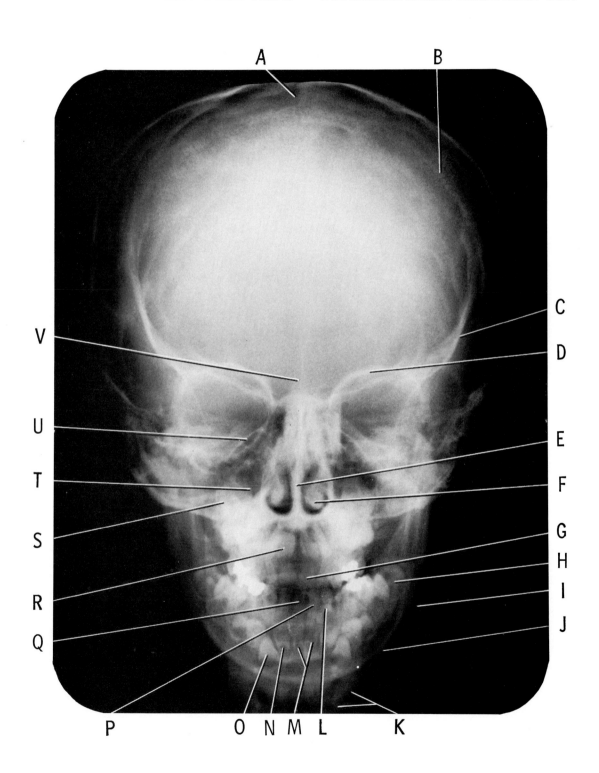

Plate 68   POSTEROANTERIOR HEADPLATE VIEW ⎯⎯⎯⎯⎯⎯⎯⎯⎯⎯⎯⎯

A.   Midsagittal suture
B.   Frontal sinus
C.   Plastic head positioner
D.   Mastoid air cells
E.   Nasal septum
F.   Nasal concha
G.   Anterior nasal spine
H.   Unerupted maxillary permanent second molar
I.   Unerupted mandibular permanent second molar
J.   Maxillary permanent central incisors
K.   Mandibular permanent central incisors
L.   Mandibular permanent lateral incisor
M.   Unerupted mandibular permanent cuspid
N.   Mandibular permanent first bicuspid
O.   Angle of mandible
P.   Neck of ramus of mandible
Q.   Maxillary sinus
R.   Petrous portion of temporal bone
S.   Orbit

Plate 68   POSTEROANTERIOR HEADPLATE VIEW

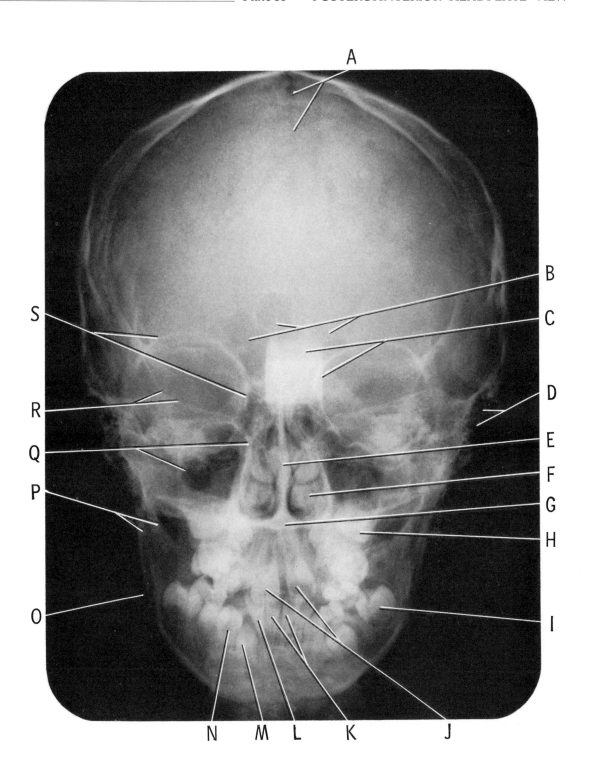

Plate 69   WATERS' SINUS HEADPLATE VIEW

A.   Frontal sinus
B.   Orbit
C.   Nasal septum
D.   Nasal conchae
E.   Maxillary sinus
F.   Zygomatic arch
G.   Anterior teeth of mandible
H.   Odontoid process of axis
I.   Foramen magnum
J.   Inferior border of mandible
K.   Posterior border of ramus of mandible
L.   Foramen rotundum

Plate 69   WATERS' SINUS HEADPLATE VIEW

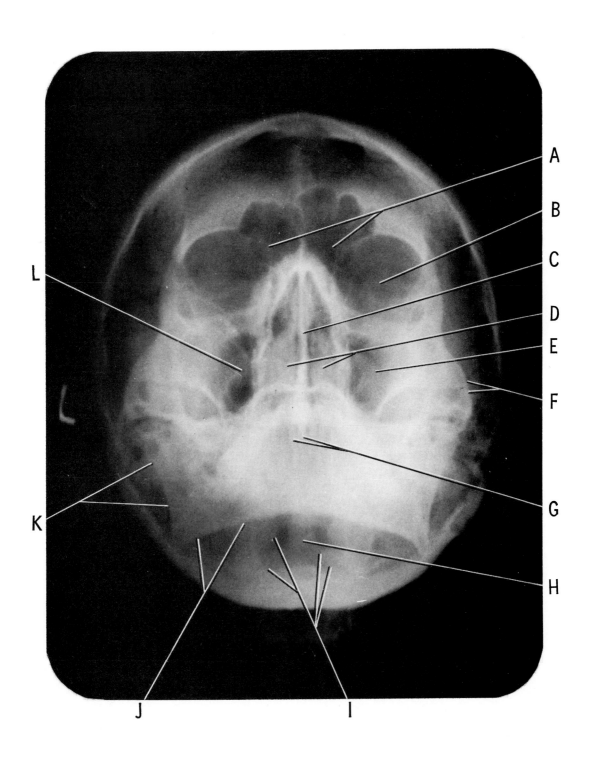

Plate 70   TEMPOROMANDIBULAR JOINT VIEW (UPDEGRAVE) _____

A. Open position
B. Rest position
C. Closed position
D. Glenoid fossa
E. Cranium interior
F. Head of mandibular condyle
G. Articular eminence
H. External auditory meatus

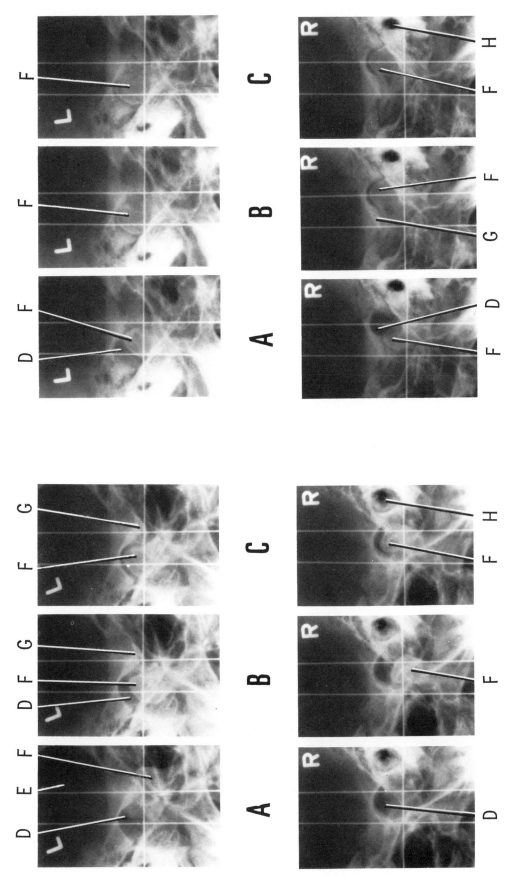

Plate 71   TEMPOROMANDIBULAR JOINT VIEW (TRANSORBITAL) _____

A.   Zygomatic arch
B.   Medial third of head of condyle
C.   Lateral third of head of condyle
D.   Neck of condyle
E.   Styloid process
F.   Mastoid process

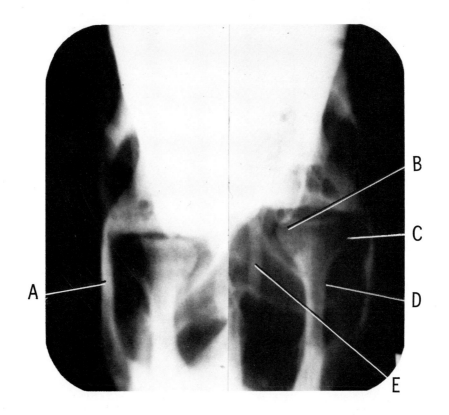

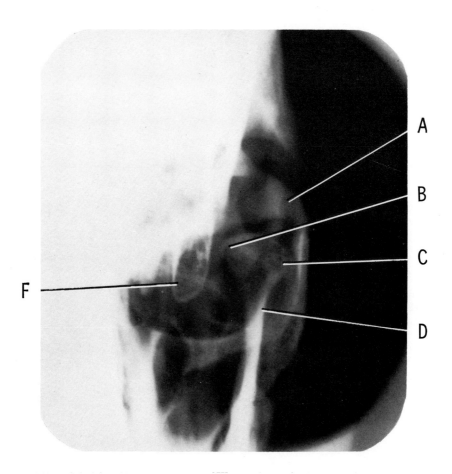

INDEX